T0208532

THE HEALTHIEST PEOPLE

THE HEALTHIEST PEOPLE
The Science behind Seventh-day Adventist Success

ELVIN ADAMS

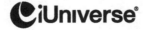

THE HEALTHIEST PEOPLE
THE SCIENCE BEHIND SEVENTH-DAY ADVENTIST SUCCESS

iUniverse books may be ordered through booksellers or by contacting:

iUniverse
1663 Liberty Drive
Bloomington, IN 47403
www.iuniverse.com
1-800-Authors (1-800-288-4677)

ISBN: 978-1-5320-9064-6 (sc)
ISBN: 978-1-5320-9065-3 (e)

Library of Congress Control Number: 2019920169

Print information available on the last page.

iUniverse rev. date: 12/12/2019

The regular pattern on the pavement of black and white stripes suggests a graph displaying regular intervals. The intervals represent various levels of health that can be achieved throughout life. People move up and down on the scale of health depending on the persistent or inconsistent application of the health choices they make.

To those who

1. *are not sick* and are free of risk factors for known diseases but who are eager to guard their health by following the practices scientifically shown to result in good health and a long life;

2. have *known risk factors* for disease and wish to reverse as far as possible the health situation they are in;

3. *suffer from disease* and want to do what they can to regain a measure of health they have lost;

4. *value science* and appreciate carefully conducted population studies with validated scientific information; and

5. are *skeptical of religion* and religious groups but who will accept results from well-designed scientific research.

CONTENTS

ACKNOWLEDGMENTS

This book would not have been possible without the expertise, experience, knowledge, encouragement, editing skills, and friendship of Judith Jamison, RD, PhD, MPH. She was intensely involved with preparing this manuscript and significantly contributed to the text.

I am indebted to Galen Bosley, DrPH, who over the period of several years meticulously found and copied every article relevant to the Adventist Health Studies. Thanks to Galen I have a hard copy of every published document related to the Adventist Health Studies.

My wife, Marie, carefully read every page and imparted a commonsense reading to complex sentences and caught all my spelling and grammatical errors. We have been married for fifty-six years.

INTRODUCTION

Health is precious. Health peaks for most people between the ages of eighteen and twenty-five. Too often it is downhill after that. You dread the decline. You get a wrinkle here and add an extra pound there. Your blood pressure creeps up along with your blood cholesterol level. Your metabolism slows down. You aren't sick, but you clearly don't have the energy you used to have.

Can anything be done? Yes, there is living among us an entire population of exceptionally healthy people. These are the Seventh-day Adventists. They are the healthiest people in the United States and probably the entire world. Adventists have less cancer and fewer heart attacks, and they enjoy overall better health and longer lives than the rest of the nation.

This isn't hype but an established fact confirmed by scientific research. Seventh-day Adventists have been studied for over seventy years. The results have been reported in more than 460 publications. The Adventist Health Studies are so important to our national health they have been largely funded by the US government. A brief history of the Adventist Health Studies is found in appendix C.

What makes Seventh-day Adventists so healthy? The earliest health proponent was a retired sea captain, Joseph Bates. He organized a temperance society in Fairhaven, Massachusetts, in 1827. He discouraged the use of tobacco, alcohol, coffee, and tea and in 1843 became a vegetarian. In the 1840s he joined the advent movement sparked by William Miller, a Baptist preacher, from which the Seventh-day Adventist Church emerged.

The foundational boost to healthful living for Seventh-day Adventists came from the writings of Ellen G. White who, in 1863, when health wasn't given much consideration by the public, laid out recommendations only recently confirmed by science. Throughout this book, quotations regarding health practices from the writings of Ellen White will occasionally be inserted to provide a sense of the accuracy of the counsel she provided the church over a hundred years ago.

Here is a sample of her counsel regarding the adequacy of a plant-based diet.

> Grains, fruits, nuts, and vegetables constitute the diet chosen for us by our Creator. These foods, prepared in as simple and natural a manner as possible, are the most healthful and nourishing. They impart a strength, a power of endurance, and a vigor of intellect that are not afforded by a more complex and stimulating diet.[1]

Ellen White concurred with Captain Bates that members should abstain from alcohol, tobacco, coffee, and tea. Additional health principles came to be known from an examination of scripture. God has placed a responsibility on each of us to care for our physical health and our spiritual well-being. The health principles developed and advocated for over 150 years have proven true. Those Seventh-day Adventists who follow the health recommendations of the church enjoy an exceptional level of good health.

Results from decades of scientific research on the health of Seventh-day Adventists are summarized in this book. Simple facts buried in complex data tables are extracted and illustrated in easy-to-read bar graphs. An orientation to the design elements used in these bar graphs is found in appendix A. Data sources are provided in detailed endnotes at the end of the book.

Are all Seventh-day Adventists healthy? No. As with any population, there are some who follow good advice and some who do not. Some who have just joined the church haven't been living a healthful lifestyle for long. Others who have been church members all their lives never embraced the health guidelines. In every group there are also those who experience limitations due to inherited diseases or serious accidents they have survived. Despite these exceptions, Seventh-day Adventists still live longer lives and have less prevalence of disease than the general public.

The bulk of the data presented here are extracted from research done at Loma Linda University in southern California on Seventh-day Adventists and can be found in articles published in peer-reviewed scientific journals. Occasionally, corroborating research conducted in secular populations will also appear in this book to support the concepts.

If you want to enjoy good health and to live a long life, this book will help you. We will focus on many lifestyle factors that promote health and longevity as proved in large human population studies. If a concept is proved on many thousands of people, then it is likely to be true for you as well.

You can experience improved health by eating healthful foods and practicing good health habits. Start building your better health now. You are invited to visit a Seventh-day Adventist church and learn of a variety of health programs they present to the community.

What is not included in this book are data from experimental studies done on laboratory animals. Information on how humans should live is primarily based on studies of humans. What is outlined here is based on established fact. It has been proved in Seventh-day Adventists. You will enjoy better health and a longer life by applying the principles provided here.

The author, Elvin Adams, is uniquely qualified to condense and present these data for your personal transformation. Helped by Galen Bosley, DrPH, the author has acquired a paper copy of every article published over the past seventy years about the health of Seventh-day Adventists. This extensive research is the primary source material for this book.

Adams has had a lifelong interest in nutrition as he was raised by parents who were vegetarians. His major field of study in college was chemistry. His medical education was obtained at the Loma Linda University School of Medicine. He is a board-certified specialist in internal medicine and for over twenty years practiced primary care in a solo office setting.

Adams pursued his interest in preventive medicine and public health at the Bloomberg School of Public Health at Johns Hopkins University, receiving a master's degree following his medical internship. He is a fellow of the American College of Preventive Medicine.

His interest and devotion to healthful living is reflected in the book he has written on obesity, *Jesus Was Thin So You Can Be Thin Too*. Dr. Adams is the creator of the Best Weigh nutrition and weight management program, which is a low-cost and often free ten-week weight loss program, usually conducted in an inexpensive church setting. Details can be viewed at BestWeigh.us.

The author is especially qualified to write about Seventh-day Adventists as he is a fifth-generation Seventh-day Adventist. Adams has served his church organization as Associate Health Ministries Director of the General Conference of Seventh-day Adventists at their world headquarters in Silver Spring, Maryland. He has also served as the Health Ministries Director of the Texas Conference of Seventh-day Adventists.

The author's understanding of the harmful effects of tobacco, alcohol, and drugs was keenly developed when he served as the medical staff director of the United States Office on Smoking and Health. In this capacity he authored one of the Surgeon General's Reports on the Health Consequences of Smoking. Since his service with the federal government, he has written or reviewed numerous articles and publications on tobacco.

After twenty-five years of clinical practice, Adams switched to the public health sector, eventually becoming the medical director and health authority for Tarrant County, Texas, where the major cities are Fort Worth and Arlington. While in this capacity, Adams became certified as a specialist in HIV/AIDS by the American Academy of HIV Medicine. He was the primary provider of services for the indigent and undocumented HIV-positive persons in a nine-county area.

Dr. Adams is almost retired. He and his wife of fifty-six years have raised three daughters. They have moved to North Carolina from Texas, where they enjoy spending time with their two young grandsons. Adams continues to write and lecture on healthful living and is actively promoting health in the community with lectures and clinics.

CHAPTER 1

Who Are the Healthiest People?

E veryone wants to be healthy. The whole nation is obsessed with health. Nobody wants to get old, sick or die. Every day we are exposed to individuals who seem especially healthy.

Health-promoting celebrities and athletes include Mehmet Oz, Oprah Winfrey, and Tom Brady. Food gurus include Mark Hyman of the Cleveland Clinic; Jenné Claiborne, a soulful vegan; and Melissa Hartwig, who is the brains behind the Whole30 program.

Then there are the fitness fanatics, including Shaun T with his *Trust and Believe* podcasts; Brittne Babe, with one million followers of her twenty-one-day challenges on Instagram; and Alexia Clark, the self-styled "Queen of Workouts."

But these are mostly fresh young faces. Will they ever grow old? Will they be physically and mentally fit in their eighties and nineties? We occasionally hear of an individual who lives to be one hundred or older. The list includes Jeanne Calment, who died at 122; Emiliano Mercado del Toro, who lived to be 115; and Besse Cooper, who survived to 116.

Unusually healthy and long-lived individuals are the exception, not the rule. You can't depend on the advice of some young, successful fitness entrepreneur. You can't depend on duplicating the experience of any centenarian just because he or she made it to one hundred or more. To be believable, you need to copy the lifestyle of a successful population—a whole group of successful people who enjoy exceptional health. Is there such a population?

Several years ago, the National Geographic staff, headed by Dan Buettner, scoured the world and found isolated pockets of people who had achieved long lives. The whole population of each area was healthy and had a concentration of people who lived to be one hundred years of age or more. These "blue zones" included Ikaria, Greece; Okinawa, Japan; Sardinia, Italy; the Nicoya Peninsula of Costa Rica; and Loma Linda, California.

The only concentration of healthy persons meeting blue zone criteria in the United States were the Seventh-day Adventists, found concentrated in Loma Linda. Seventh-day Adventists are the healthiest people in this country. Adventists are not only found in southern California; more than a million are scattered across the land, and there are over twenty million Seventh-day Adventists in two hundred countries all around the world.

There is a mini blue zone in every Seventh-day Adventist church. The health of Seventh-day Adventists was not discovered by Dan Buettner. Adventists have been promoting health since the 1840s. Seventh-day Adventists have been the object of large population studies since the 1950s.

The health of Seventh-day Adventists has been carefully documented in hundreds of peer-reviewed scientific papers published in the major scientific journals of the world. The scientific community has largely come to understand Seventh-day Adventists enjoy better health and live longer than any other population group in the United States.

The object of this book is to take the mountain of scientific facts written about the health of Seventh-day Adventists and to distill important points into easy-to-understand words and images that will be informative and motivate you to live a more healthful lifestyle.

The largest population study of Seventh-day Adventists is called the Adventist Health Study II (AHS-II). It includes nearly one hundred thousand Adventists from Loma Linda and church populations across the United States and Canada. (See appendix C for an expanded history of AHS research.)

One of the major focuses of the study was the diet of Seventh-day Adventists. Not all Adventists eat the same. Because of the large size of the population, it is possible to subdivide the study population by differences in the diet.[1] Five diet categories are described. AHS-II research compares different diet groups within the Adventist population.

Diet Category 1: Non-vegetarian Seventh-day Adventists

The largest diet category of Seventh-day Adventists is the non-vegetarian. This group comprises 43.7 percent of the study population and eats all foods, including fruits, vegetables, dairy products, fish, poultry, and red meat. These Adventists with the most liberal diet are the least healthy segment of our population.

Some of these individuals are new converts to the church and haven't fully adopted the dietary practices of more health-conscious Seventh-day Adventists. Others are established church members who just haven't subscribed to the health principles of the church. Still, this non-vegetarian group is consuming less meat, poultry, and fish than people who are not Seventh-day Adventists.

Despite these variations, Seventh-day Adventists are significantly healthier than their neighbors and friends who live in the same community. The AHS-II study does not compare the health experience of each diet category of Seventh-day Adventists with that of non-Adventists, but the health of each of the diet categories is measured against the health of non-vegetarian Seventh-day Adventists.

Diet Category 2: Semi-vegetarian
Seventh-day Adventists

The second diet category is the semi-vegetarian. This group of Seventh-day Adventists eats all food categories but very little fish, poultry, and red meat. Only 8.3 percent of the population falls into this category. The health of these Seventh-day Adventists is better than that of the non-vegetarian group.

Diet Category 3: Pesco-vegetarian Seventh-day Adventists

The third diet group of Seventh-day Adventists is the pesco-vegetarian. These people do not eat meat or poultry but do eat fish as well as dairy products and fruits and vegetables. Only 9.7 percent of Seventh-day Adventists fall into this group. The health of this group is better than those who include poultry and red meat in the diet.

Diet Category 4: Lacto-ovo Vegetarian Seventh-day Adventists

This group does not eat fish, poultry, or red meat but does include dairy products in their diet. They eat eggs, milk, cheese, yogurt, butter, ice cream, and all other dairy products. This is the second largest group of Seventh-day Adventists, comprising 34 percent of the study population. The health of this group is better than those who include fish, poultry, and red meat in their diet.

Diet Category 5: Vegan Vegetarian Seventh-day Adventists

This group's diet consists entirely of plant-based foods. They avoid fish, poultry, red meat, and all dairy products. This is the smallest diet group of Seventh-day Adventists, comprising just 4.3 percent of the study population. They enjoy the best level of health.

The dietary practices of these five diet categories are summarized in figure 1.

Figure 1. Five diet categories of Seventh-day Adventists and the types of foods consumed by each group[2]

Five Diet Categories of Seventh-day Adventists					
Category	Percent of Population	Fruits & Vegetables	Milk, Eggs, & Cheese	Fish	Poultry & Red Meat
Non-Vegetarian	43.7%	Yes	Yes	Yes	Yes
Semi-Vegetarian	8.3%	Yes	Yes	Some	Some
Pesco-Vegetarian	9.7%	Yes	Yes	Yes	No
Lacto-Ovo Vegetarian	34.0%	Yes	Yes	No	No
Vegan	4.3%	Yes	No	No	No

Diet and Disease Relationships

The five diet categories of Seventh-day Adventists result in various levels of disease and risk factors for disease. Diabetes has become a major cause of morbidity and mortality in the United States and the world. People with diabetes are at increased risk of many complications, which are mainly due to high blood sugar levels, insulin resistance, chronic continuous low-grade inflammation, and rapidly developing hardening of the arteries throughout the body.

Diabetics have an elevated risk of heart attacks, strokes, and heart failure. Kidney failure has many causes, but diabetes is a major risk factor. Disease of the retina of the eye is a risk factor for reduced vision and blindness. Diseased nerves and blood vessels lead to painful yet numb extremities, foot ulcers, and, frequently, amputations of toes, feet, or legs. Diabetes increases the risk of some cancers. Deteriorating mental status, sleep apnea, and mood disorders are also complications of diabetes.[3]

The risk of diabetes in Seventh-day Adventists is highest in the non-vegetarian diet group. The level of diabetes in this group may be the same or lower than in the general population. This has not been determined. If the rate of diabetes in the non-vegetarian Seventh-day Adventists is set to 1, then the prevalence of diabetes decreases in each dietary group of Seventh-day Adventists as their diet moves toward the vegan diet. The vegan Seventh-day Adventists experience only 22 percent of the diabetes of the non-vegetarian group.[4]

Figure 2. Risk of diabetes in Seventh-day Adventists by the five diet categories Significance p = 0.0001[5]

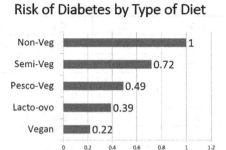

Dramatic results are also seen for the risk of high blood pressure by dietary group. High blood pressure usually has no symptoms but is a major risk factor for heart attacks, heart failure, strokes, chronic kidney disease, eye damage, blockage in arteries and legs, aneurysms, and dementia due to blockage of blood vessels in the brain.[6]

The prevalence of high blood pressure varies dramatically in Seventh-day Adventists in different diet categories.[7] High blood pressure is highest in the non-vegetarian group. The vegan Seventh-day Adventists have only a quarter of the high blood pressure compared to the non-vegetarian group.

Figure 3. The prevalence of high blood pressure in Seventh-day Adventists by the five diet categories Significance p = 0.0001[8]

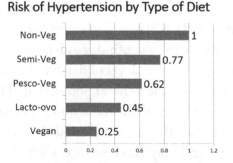

Diet also has a significant effect on a person's weight. In scientific research, relative weight is measured by the body mass index (BMI). Normal weight is defined as a BMI between 18 and 24.9. The overweight category is defined as a BMI between 25 and 29.9. Obesity begins with a BMI of 30 and goes up from there.

Obesity has become a global public health issue. In some states, more than 35 percent of adults over the age of eighteen are obese.[9] When the overweight category is added to the obese category, there are many states where 66 percent of the population is overweight or obese. Sadly, no state or country has ever successfully reduced the prevalence of obesity in its territory over the last thirty-three years.[10]

Obesity varies by denomination and church affiliation. Baptists, Fundamentalist Protestant denominations, and Catholics weigh more than members of other denominations. The Seventh-day Adventists, Mormons, and Jehovah's Witnesses are the denominations with the least obesity.[11]

Among Seventh-day Adventists, obesity varies by dietary group.[12] None of the groups had weights in the obese category of a BMI over 30. The heaviest group of Seventh-day Adventists is the non-vegetarian, with an average BMI of 28.3. The average BMI of the vegans was 23.1. The vegans as a group were the only normal-weight group of Seventh-day Adventists.

Figure 4. The distribution of weight by BMI of Seventh-day Adventists by the five diet types[13]

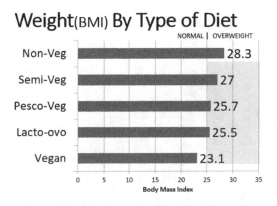

Seventh-day Adventist vegans are the healthiest group of people in the United States and the world, but these figures demonstrate there are dramatic differences among Adventists by the type of diet adhered to. We will be looking in detail at the quantity of specific food items eaten by the five diet categories and discover the health benefits that result from specific foods and categories of food.

CHAPTER 2

Why the Healthiest People Live Longer

The most fundamental and possibly the best measure of the health of a population is life expectancy. Life expectancy is the average age at which half the people are dead, and the other half are still alive. Naturally, life expectancy is different for men and women. One of the best ways to measure the health of any group of people is to examine their life expectancy.

Life expectancy varies widely from country to country.[1] Life expectancy at birth in Japan is 84.74 years; Switzerland, 82.5; Canada, 81.76; Germany, 80.57; and the United States, 79.68 years. The United States ranks number forty-three in life expectancy among the other large and small countries of the world. The worst country, at number 224, is Chad, with a life expectancy of only 49.81 years.

Life expectancy in the United States is slowly decreasing. On average, the life expectancy for someone born in 2015 fell from 78.9 years to 78.8 years. The life expectancy for the average American man fell two-tenths of a year—from 76.5 to 76.3. For women, it dropped one-tenth—from 81.3 to 81.2 years.[2]

All the health gains the United States benefited from by discouraging smoking, controlling blood pressure, lowering cholesterol, and improving automobile safety are slowly being undone. The epidemic of obesity and associated diseases and deaths from drug overdoses are chipping away at the nation's health.

There has also been an increase in the number of deaths from eight of the top ten causes in the United States. Deaths from heart disease and stroke are going up after going down for years. Deaths are also increasing from Alzheimer's disease, emphysema, kidney disease, diabetes, injuries, and suicide.

The primary goal of healthful living is to extend life expectancy. This can be done by following the principles laid out in this book. God wants you to live the abundant life and enjoy good health. Jesus said, "I have come that they may have *life*, and that they may have it *more abundantly*" (John 10:10). (See appendix E for more Bible references to health.)

The Adventist Health Studies-I were conducted at Loma Linda, California, and examined the life expectancy of Seventh-day Adventists compared to the life expectancy of California contemporaries. Figure 1 is a graph showing the life expectancy of Seventh-day Adventist men by decade of life.[3]

Figure 1. Life expectancy of Seventh-day Adventist men in California compared to other matched California males who were part of an American Cancer Society study population[4]

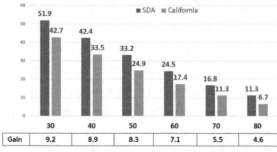

Life Expectancy of SDA and California Males by Decade

	30	40	50	60	70	80
Gain	9.2	8.9	8.3	7.1	5.5	4.6

Life expectancy for US men at birth is 76.3 years. By age thirty men have lived thirty years and so have a shorter remaining life expectancy. In this graph we compare the life expectancy of Seventh-day Adventist men living in California with carefully matched California men of the same age, race, place of residence, and so on. At age thirty, Seventh-day Adventist men have on average 51.9 years of life left to live, while other California men can only expect to live 42.7 more years. That is an amazing 9.2-year advantage for Seventh-day Adventist men.

Notice that at every decade of life, Seventh-day Adventist men have several more years of life remaining compared to other men living in the same community. Even at age eighty, Seventh-day Adventist men live five and a half years longer than their neighbors of identical age.

This longevity advantage is because Seventh-day Adventist men are healthy. They have less heart disease, less cancer, and less of most every disease—so they live longer. The rest of this book looks at specific things that give Seventh-day Adventists this advantage.

Figure 2 shows that the results are similar for Seventh-day Adventist women based on the same study.

Figure 2. Life expectancy of Seventh-day Adventist females in California compared to other matched California females who were part of an American Cancer Society study population[5]

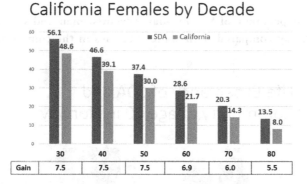

Life Expectancy of SDA and California Females by Decade

| Gain | 7.5 | 7.5 | 7.5 | 6.9 | 6.0 | 5.5 |

Seventh-day Adventist women living in California at age thirty will live on average 56.1 more years, compared with only 48.6 years for other women in California.

First, notice that Seventh-day Adventist women at every decade of life live longer than Seventh-day Adventist men. At age thirty, Adventist men in figure 1 will live 51.9 more years, while Adventist women at age thirty will live on average 56.1 more years. In the United States, women live longer than men, and this is true among Seventh-day Adventists as well.

Second, notice that at age thirty, the years gained over contemporaries for women is 7.5 years, while it is 9.2 years for men. This difference is primarily due to differences in cigarette smoking between men and women.

At the time of this study, California women didn't smoke nearly as much as California men. That made them basically healthier than men to begin with. So when comparing nonsmoking California women with Seventh-day Adventist women, the difference is as not as great as in men.

Seventh-day Adventists have one million members in the United States and comprise a global church with over twenty million members. Seventh-day Adventists have been studied in several other countries and continue to show a significant advantage in life expectancy over their contemporaries.

For example, in Norway, Seventh-day Adventists have an advantage in life expectancy.[6] The advantage is 5.2 years for both men and women.

Figure 3. Life expectancy of Seventh-day Adventist men and women at age twenty in Norway compared with contemporaries in the community of the same age[7]

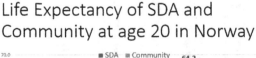

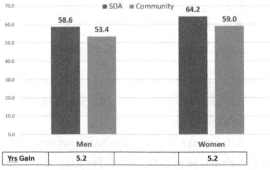

In the Netherlands, Seventh-day Adventists have a life expectancy advantage at age twenty-seven of 8.9 years for men and 4.6 years for women.[8]

Figure 4. Life expectancy of Seventh-day Adventist men and women at age twenty-seven in the Netherlands compared with contemporary community members of the same age[9]

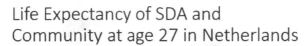
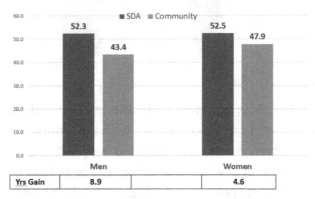

Life Expectancy of SDA and Community at age 27 in Netherlands

Concepts similar to life expectancy are *overall mortality* and the *standardized mortality ratio*. In these calculations, the total of all causes of death for one group is compared with the total of all causes of death for another group.

An exceptionally large study of mortality was done in Japan.[10] This study included 122,261 men forty years of age and older in both urban and rural settings followed for sixteen years. Over this time period, 5,132 deaths occurred. This population was divided into various groups depending on several factors, including meat in the diet, consumption of green and yellow vegetables, alcohol consumption, and cigarette smoking.

The healthiest people in this study turned out to be Seventh-day Adventists and others with a lifestyle like Seventh-day Adventists. The healthiest people did not eat meat, did not drink alcoholic beverages, and did not smoke, but they did eat green and yellow vegetables daily.

Figure 5. Mortality ratio for all causes of death of Seventh-day Adventist men ages forty and older compared to Japanese men in the same age category who were not Seventh-day Adventists[11]

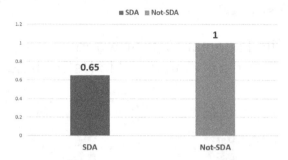

Mortality Ratio of Japanese Men 40 and Older

Seventh-day Adventist men had mortality from all causes only 65 percent of that of those Japanese men with the unhealthiest lifestyle. Seventh-day Adventists are the healthiest people living in Japan.

A small study of Seventh-day Adventists in Poland indicates that Seventh-day Adventists live much longer than their contemporaries.[12]

The earlier in life one becomes a Seventh-day Adventist, the longer one can expect to experience a longer life and reduced deaths from several causes.[13]

Ellen White equated long life to results from adherence to the laws of nature.

> Intellectual power, physical stamina, and *length of life* depend upon immutable laws. Nature's God will not interfere to preserve men from the consequences of violating nature's requirements. He who strives for the mastery must be temperate in all things.[14]

Lifestyle Elements That Affect Life Expectancy and Overall Mortality

Nutrition

Among the predictive factors of successful aging, nutrition is one of the major determinants. The dynamics of nutrition will be the primary focus of this book. Excellent nutrition helps maintain physical and mental functioning. Inadequate nutrition contributes to losing function and to the promotion and progression of disease.

Many scientific findings indicate the close relationship between nutrition and longevity. One list of ten foods and promote longevity includes the following.[15]

1. Cruciferous vegetables
2. Salad greens
3. Nuts
4. Seeds
5. Berries
6. Pomegranate
7. Beans
8. Mushrooms
9. Onions and garlic
10. Tomatoes

While a good diet does not guarantee freedom from disease and longevity, it will provide a stronger immune system and increased strength and vitality and can minimize inflammation, which is one of the worst offenders in aging. Inflammation is a factor in many of the chronic diseases that cause most early deaths.

Obesity

Another important determining factor of life expectancy is obesity. Not only what is eaten but also the amount eaten is important. A recent study showed that severe obesity cut life expectancy by up to ten years. The findings contradict earlier evidence of an "obesity paradox," which indicated that overweight people did not die sooner. This recent study found that moderately overweight people lost about a year of life expectancy on the average, but that mortality soared in those with more serious weight problems.[16]

The National Cancer Institute recently analyzed twenty large studies of people from three countries. They found that people with class III (extreme obesity) had a dramatic reduction in life expectancy compared with people of normal weight. Years of life lost ranged from 6.5 years to 13.7 years.[17] This topic will be covered in greater detail in another chapter.

Today many books and videos illustrate that often our graves are dug with the fork. America is not the healthiest nation. Proper food choices must be made daily. Today's food is processed and engineered with sometimes harmful items added that offer little nutritional value. Vigilance is needed every day to promote long, disease-free lives.

Positive Attitude and Longevity

Embracing a positive attitude is yet another factor affecting longevity. Factors that contribute to attaining a positive attitude include the following:

1. Maintain an attitude of gratitude. Take inventory of your life and count the good things around you and give God praise and thanksgiving for his abundant goodness toward you.
2. Have a firm, strong, bounce-back composure instead of grumbling and complaining. Resiliency is staying calm and weathering the storm with a smile on your face.
3. Accept life as it is, and don't wish for something that has not or will not happen. Accept yourself and others with a positive, cheerful attitude.
4. Take a laugh break. Watching fifteen minutes of a funny video or TV can improve blood flow to your heart by 50 percent.

This may reduce blood-clot formation, cholesterol deposition, and inflammation. [18]

5. Leave off the worrying. Constant worrying may shorten your life span.

6. Cultivate an optimistic attitude. A study done at the Mayo Clinic on 839 patients found those who were more pessimistic experienced a 19 percent increase in the risk of dying. [19]

In another study of 660 participants, it was found that people having a positive attitude lived 7.5 years longer than their contemporaries. This effect remained even after other factors, such as age, gender, income, and loneliness, influencing health status were controlled for. [20]

People with positive attitudes produce lower levels of stress hormones, which help protect them from disease. Researchers have found that people with a positive attitude during stressful events are 22 percent less likely to have a fatal or nonfatal heart attack than those who have negative attitudes. [21]

Ellen White connected a positive attitude with health and a long life.

> Courage, hope, faith, sympathy, love, promote health and prolong life. A contented mind, a cheerful spirit, is health to the body and strength to the soul. "A merry [rejoicing] heart doeth good like a medicine" (Proverbs 17:22). [22]

Other Factors Affecting Longevity

Cigarette smoking is the most important cause of premature disease and death. Cigarette smoking causes 155,000 lung cancer deaths in the United States each year. [23] Lung cancer is the number one cause of death in both men and women. Totaling all the premature deaths among men and women in the United States caused by smoking each year, the total reaches 480,000. [24] The greatest habit/addiction that lowers life expectancy is cigarette smoking. Alcohol and drugs lower life expectancy to a lesser degree than the adverse effects of tobacco.

Regular endurance exercise keeps muscles strong, fights depression, and adds years to your life. Exposure to sunshine in moderate amounts boosts vitamin D levels and improves mood. Adequate rest, breathing in clean, fresh air, and trust in God's loving, sustaining care all contribute to a long and healthy life.

Summary

The average life expectancy is only about 28,105 days (77 years). Improved daily food choices are a must to extend those years. And research has shown that we can do it!

The February 20, 2009, issue of *U.S News and World Reports*[25] outlined eleven recommendations to live to be one hundred. Shown here is their number eight recommendation. This should be the best outline for success in living a long and full life.

> 8. *Live like a Seventh Day Adventist.* Americans who define themselves as Seventh-day Adventists have an average life expectancy of 89, about a decade longer than the average American. One of the basic tenets of the religion is that it's important to cherish the body that's on loan from God, which means no smoking, alcohol abuse, or overindulging in sweets. Followers typically stick to a vegetarian diet based on fruits, vegetables, beans, and nuts, and get plenty of exercise. They're also very focused on family and community.

This book provides an in-depth look into the diet of Seventh-day Adventists and the impact food plays in making them the healthiest group of people in the United States and the world.

Socrates once stated, "Bad men live that they may eat and drink, whereas good men eat and drink that they may live."[26] There is much truth in that statement.

God outlined for us his health guidelines in the Bible. Because he created us, he knew what would be best to promote health and longevity. God wants us to live long, quality-filled years. God wants us to be happy and free from disease. From the beginning he instituted a diet, an exercise program, proper rest, and relaxation where health could flourish and life could be enjoyed. Following these biblical guidelines, we today can also live life to its fullness. (See appendix E for additional references.)

CHAPTER 3

Fabulous Citrus Fruit

Fruits of all kinds contribute to good health. The eating of various types of fruit by Seventh-day Adventists has been documented in the Adventist Health Study.[1] The vegans and pesco-vegetarian Adventists consume the most fruit. The least amount of fruit is consumed by the non-vegetarian Seventh-day Adventists. Fruit in the diet is a major contributor to the exceptional good health enjoyed by the healthiest Seventh-day Adventists.

Figure 1. The daily average consumption of fruit in grams per day by Seventh-day Adventists in five different diet categories in the United States[2]

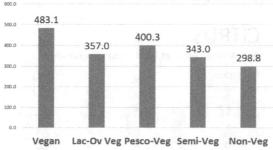

All FRUIT
Daily Average Eating of Food Groups in Grams/day

Vegan: 483.1
Lac-Ov Veg: 357.0
Pesco-Veg: 400.3
Semi-Veg: 343.0
Non-Veg: 298.8

Ellen White encouraged the church membership to eat more fruit, especially fresh fruit.

> It would be well for us to do less cooking and to eat more fruit in its natural state. Let us teach the people to eat freely of the fresh grapes, apples, peaches, pears, berries, and all other kinds of fruit that can be obtained. Let these be prepared for winter use by canning, using glass, as far as possible, instead of tin.[3]

There are different kinds of fruit, and each category possesses unique health-enhancing qualities. We begin by focusing on citrus.

Citrus is native to South and East Asia. References to citrus have been found in Chinese literature as early as 2000 BC. Citrus fruit references in Europe date from 300 BC. Citrus was introduced to the Americas by Columbus and Ponce de Léon in the 1500s. Citrus fruits have long been appreciated as part of a nourishing and tasty diet. Oranges, grapefruit, lemons, and limes are the citrus with the largest commercial value and are sold worldwide.

Citrus fruits have wonderful health-enhancing qualities. The use of citrus fruit by the five diet categories of Seventh-day Adventists is presented here. The healthiest Adventists consume 40 percent more citrus per day than the least healthy Adventists.

Figure 2. The daily average consumption of citrus fruit in grams per day by Seventh-day Adventists in five diet categories[4]

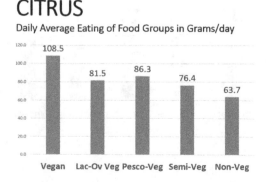

CITRUS
Daily Average Eating of Food Groups in Grams/day

Cancer and Citrus

Prostate Cancer and Citrus

In the Adventist Health Study, citrus was found to dramatically reduce the risk of prostate cancer. In this portion of the study, fourteen thousand men were followed for seven years.[5] Here are the results.

Figure 3. Prostate cancer by the amount of fresh citrus fruit in the diet of 14,000 SDA men followed from 1976 to 1982[6]
Significance p = 0.008

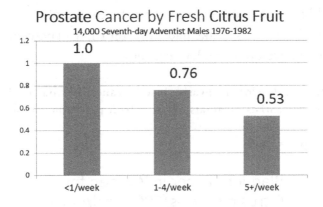

For men eating citrus one to four times a week, the risk of dying from prostate cancer was reduced 24 percent. The results were nearly twice as good for men eating citrus five or more times a week. These men experienced a 47 percent reduction in the risk of death from prostate cancer.

This study of Adventist men was published in 1989. More recent advances in the diagnosis and treatment of prostate cancer have improved outcomes to some extent. As of this writing, prostate cancer is the most commonly diagnosed cancer in men and the third leading cause of cancer deaths after cancers of the lung and colon. The American Cancer Society estimates there are 161,000 new cases of prostate cancer diagnosed each year, and there are 26,700 deaths from prostate cancer.[7] This indicates that prostate cancer continues to be a significant health problem.

Bladder Cancer and Citrus

In the United States, in women, there are about 18,500 new cases and 4,600 deaths from bladder cancer each year. Factors that can be avoided that contribute to bladder cancer include cigarette smoking, exposure to certain chemicals in industrial settings, and taking the diabetes medication pioglitazone (Actos).[8] The regular intake of citrus will reduce the risk of developing bladder cancer.

A study of bladder cancer in a population of over one hundred thousand women who were not Seventh-day Adventists, followed for several years, found that the risk of developing invasive bladder cancer was steadily diminished by increasing the intake of citrus.[9] Women with the highest citrus intake had a greater than 50 percent reduction in the risk of developing bladder cancer.

Figure 4. Risk of developing invasive bladder cancer in women who were not Seventh-day Adventists by grams of citrus fruit per 1,000 calories consumed per day[10]
Significance p = <0.001

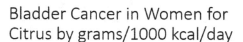

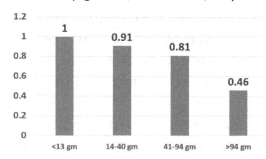

Fruit juice was not nearly as effective as eating fruit itself. In this same study, only the women with the highest intake of fruit juice were benefited with reduced bladder cancer risk. This benefit was not statistically significant.

Figure 5. Risk of developing invasive bladder cancer in women who were not Seventh-day Adventists by grams of citrus juice per 1,000 calories consumed per day[11]
Significance p = 0.05

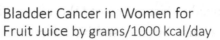
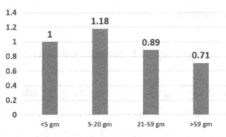

Bladder Cancer in Women for
Fruit Juice by grams/1000 kcal/day

Breast Cancer and Citrus

In a large case-control study of breast cancer in Shanghai, China, citrus fruits were found to reduce the risk of breast cancer. In this study there were 3,443 cases of breast cancer and 3,474 controls without breast cancer.[12] Although this study compared results among women whose breast tumors were positive or negative for estrogen receptors and progesterone receptors, the benefit was across the board and not specific for one group of women with a unique receptor combination.

Figure 6. Breast cancer risk of Chinese women who were not Seventh-day Adventists by the amount of citrus in the diet per day. A case-control study.[13]
Significance p = 0.003

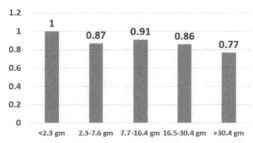

Breast Cancer Risk
by grams/day of Citrus in the Diet

The diagnosis and treatment of breast cancer is improving steadily in the United States. Breast cancer is the most commonly diagnosed cancer, with over two hundred fifty thousand new cases a year. Fortunately, due to advances in treatment, the number of deaths per year has been reduced to just over forty thousand. The regular intake of citrus can have a small but measurable effect in reducing the risk of developing breast cancer.

Esophageal Cancer and Citrus

Cancer of the esophagus is increasing in the United States and around the world. In the United States, there are nearly seventeen thousand new cases each year and over fifteen thousand deaths. Worldwide there are over four hundred fifty thousand new cases each year. Cancer of the esophagus is the sixth most common cause of cancer death.[14] Risk factors for developing esophageal cancer include smoking tobacco in any form, drinking alcohol, obesity, drinking hot liquids, and having bile reflux into the esophagus from the stomach.[15]

A large meta-analysis of the relationship between citrus intake and cancer of the esophagus included data from nineteen studies conducted in the United States, Italy, Japan, France, Europe, China, Argentina, Switzerland, Uruguay, and the Netherlands. Overall, the addition of citrus in the diet reduced the risk of dying from esophageal cancer by 37 percent.[16]

Figure 7. Risk of developing esophageal cancer for several hundred thousand men and women in a meta-analysis of multiple studies conducted in North and South America, Europe, and Asia who are not Seventh-day Adventists by including citrus in the diet compared with those who did not eat citrus[17] Significance p = 0.0001

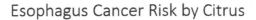

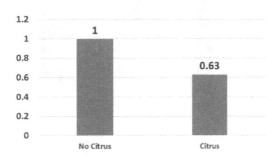

Esophagus Cancer Risk by Citrus

Lung cancer is the number one cause of cancer deaths in both men and women in the United States, responsible for over eighty-four thousand deaths per year in men and over seventy-one thousand deaths per year in women. Cigarette smoking is the only major cause of lung cancer. While several dietary factors have been identified that can reduce the risk of lung cancer in smokers, we will only look at the reduction in risk imparted by citrus.

Lung Cancer and Citrus

The Pooling project includes data from eight large prospective studies including 280,419 women and 149,862 men. During the study, 3,206 cases of lung cancer developed, divided nearly equally between men and women. As smokers ate more oranges and tangerines, they experienced less lung cancer.[18] Those who ate up to one serving per week had an 18 percent reduction in lung cancer, and those who ate from one serving per week to one-half serving per day experienced a 26 percent reduction in lung cancer compared with those who ate no citrus.

Figure 8. Risk of developing lung cancer for men and women who are not Seventh-day Adventists by the amount of citrus in the diet[19]
Significance p = 0.006

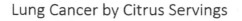
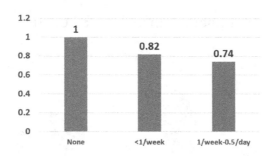

Lung Cancer by Citrus Servings

Heart Disease and Citrus

Coronary heart disease is the number one cause of death in the United States. For persons under the age of sixty-five, cancer is the leading cause of death; but for older Americans, heart disease edges out cancer, becoming the leading cause of death.

In younger citizens, men have more heart attacks than women; but in older citizens, heart attacks in women exceed those for men. There are more women alive than men in older age groups. In the latest year for which exact numbers are available, there were 614,348 deaths from heart diseases and 591,699 deaths from cancers.[20]

Heart disease is affected by multiple risk factors[21]—many of which can be modified by changes in lifestyle. Major risk factors include the following:

1. High blood pressure
2. High blood cholesterol
3. Smoking
4. Diabetes and prediabetes
5. Overweight and obesity
6. Physical inactivity

7. Family history of heart disease
8. History of blood pressure problems during pregnancy
9. Unhealthy diet
10. Age

Many different foods decrease the risk of developing heart disease. One category is citrus. One large study that specifically looked at citrus and heart disease used data from the Nurses' Health Study, which followed 71,141 women, and the Health Professionals Follow-up Study, which included 42,135 men. During these studies, 2,582 heart events occurred in women, and 3,607 heart events occurred in men.

In this study, the benefits of including fruits and vegetables in the diet were documented.[22] This graph illustrates the benefit of eating citrus for women.

Figure 9. Risk of coronary heart disease for women who are not Seventh-day Adventists by the average amount of citrus servings per day.[23]
Significance p = <0.0001

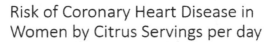

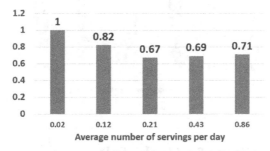

Risk of Coronary Heart Disease in Women by Citrus Servings per day

The maximum benefit occurred with a low intake of citrus and then leveled off. The maximum benefit was met with just 0.21 servings per day on average. This is equal to one and a half servings of citrus per week. Increasing this by a factor of two or four provided no additional benefit by further reducing the risk of heart disease.

This is still a significant benefit. With just moderate citrus intake, women reduced the risk of heart attacks by 33 percent. Citrus is very protective and significantly reduces the risk of heart attacks. Additional benefits can be realized by stopping smoking, controlling blood pressure, maintaining a normal weight, and exercising regularly, but adding citrus to the diet is a powerful way to reduce the risk of having or dying from a heart attack.

The results for men were not as dramatic. Men eating an average of 0.2 servings per day (one and a half servings per week) had a 16 percent reduction in the risk of heart attacks, which held steady. Even if a man ate citrus every day of the week, there was no further improvement in heart attack risk.

Figure 10. Risk of coronary heart disease for men who are not Seventh-day Adventists by the average amount of citrus servings per day.[24] Significance p = <0.005

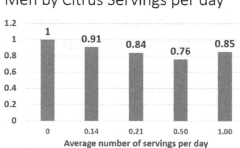

What Makes Citrus So Healthful?

The exact mechanisms by which citrus results in health benefits have not been fully determined. Citrus is an excellent source of vitamins, minerals, and complex phytochemicals. Take your nutrition directly from the whole food and do not focus on specific chemicals found in foods.

One factor in citrus fruits that contributes to lowering the risk of heart disease is that citrus contains high levels of folate. Folate lowers the homocysteine level in the blood, which injures the lining of the blood vessels, contributing to heart disease. In addition, citrus is high in vitamin C, which acts as an antioxidant to quench harmful free radicals that can damage the delicate lining of blood vessels.

Citrus is known for its many other protective effects besides its antioxidant, anticancer, and cardiovascular protection. Citrus has potent anti-inflammatory and neuroprotective properties. Citrus can also prevent chronic nerve damage resulting from diabetes or celiac disease.

Citrus is best known for the high levels of vitamin C it contains. But it is also a good source for many of the B vitamins. Vitamin C plays many roles in the body, such as it increases the absorption of iron, protects the eyes against cataracts, increases bone mineral density, reduces kidney stones, and is even thought to play a role in increasing cognition in the elderly.

In addition, citrus is an excellent source of many minerals, such as potassium, phosphorus, calcium, magnesium, and copper. And as an added benefit, citrus contains many phytochemicals that work in synergy with one another to reduce the risk of chronic diseases. Some of these include monoterpenes, limonoids, flavonoids, carotenoids and hydroxycinnamic acid.[25]

Fresh whole citrus fruits are a good source of dietary fiber. One medium orange contains three grams of soluble fiber. This nonglycemic fiber can form a gel-like matrix that can slow the absorption of glucose, delay gastric emptying time, and prevent blood sugar spikes. Therefore, whole fruit is recommended versus fruit juice.

Certain groups of people especially benefit from a high citrus consumption. They are smokers, alcoholics, patients with severe burns, fractures, fever, tuberculosis, post-surgery, critically ill, immunocompromised individuals, children, and the elderly.

Do We Eat Enough Citrus?

US fresh citrus fruit consumption per capita has remained essentially flat over the past fifteen years at twenty-two pounds of citrus per person per year.[26] Translated into grams, this averages out to be 9,988g/year or 192g/week. Put into cups, this would equal 1 cup/week or one-eighth cup per day. This is far below recommended levels. This statistic is based on pounds of total fruit, including the peel, not the edible portion only.

While there is no established dietary recommendation for citrus fruits, it is generally felt that four or five servings/week is adequate. For special vulnerable groups of people, more would be required.

There are over fifty varieties of citrus fruits, with over one hundred more counting all the hybrids. Some of the common ones are oranges, mandarins (including clementines, halos, cuties, and tangerines), grapefruit, tangelo, lemons, and limes, and some uncommon ones such as satsuma, kumquat, and calamondin. They are literally grown all around the world.

Brazil is the top producer of oranges, where China and the United States produce the most tangerines and grapefruit respectively. India produces the most lemons and limes. Citrus fruit is available the year round through importation and locally grown in California, Texas, and Florida.

How can we incorporate citrus in our diet? Usually this is not a problem as the fruit comes ready-to-eat. Oranges and tangerines can simply be peeled, and the segments of fruit easily eaten. However, citrus segments can be used in salads, fruit compotes, squeezed as fresh juice, and even in some entrees in Asian cuisine.

Some are deceived into thinking that real citrus is found in many beverages, drinks, popsicles, gelatin, yogurt, and candy with orange or lemon in the name. Artificially flavored food items have none of the health benefits real citrus can provide.

You might want to try the citrus recipes included in this book in order to add a wider variety of citrus fruits to your diet. Lemon pie and lemonade are two highly desirable citrus foods, but they can be high in sugar. Recipes for a sugar-free smoothie can be made to replace sugar-laden lemonade, and a sugar-free lemon pie recipe is provided that can serve as a tasty substitute.

Recipes

Orange Smoothie—serves 2

1 medium orange, peeled and seeded
1/2 cup orange juice
1 cup soymilk
2/3 cup ice cubes
1 small banana or 1/2 cup peeled mango chunks
1 teaspoon vanilla extract

Place all ingredients in a blender and process until smooth. Divide in two glasses. Garnish with a slice of orange.

Citrus Salad—serves 7

2 (5-ounce) bags of mixed salad greens
1 large avocado, cubed
1 cup Ruby Red grapefruit sections
1 cup orange sections or 1 (8-ounce) can mandarin oranges
orange poppy seed dressing to taste
20 toasted walnut halves

Lightly toss together the salad greens, avocado, and the fruit and divide on seven plates. Drizzle orange poppy seed dressing over each salad and garnish with the walnuts.

Ambrosia—serves 4

4 medium oranges, peeled and sliced

1/2 cup shredded coconut
2 tablespoons pistachio nuts or pomegranate seeds

Divide oranges on four plates.
Sprinkle coconut on the top.
Garnish with pistachio nuts or pomegranate seeds.
Optional: Fresh pineapple chunks and/or red grapes can be added if desired.

Lemon Pie—serves 6

4 cups pineapple juice
1/2 cup fresh lemon juice
2/3 cup cornstarch
1/2 cup honey
1 cup fresh or frozen raspberries or blueberries
1 graham cracker crust or prebaked pie crust
1 container dairy-free whipped topping
lemon, thinly sliced

Whisk together the pineapple juice, lemon juice, cornstarch, and honey. Bring to a boil, stirring constantly until well thickened. Remove from heat. Place berries on prepared crust; pour warm lemon mixture over berries. Refrigerate until well set. Top with dairy-free whipped topping and garnish with lemon slices.

CHAPTER 4

Apples, Pears, Berries, and Dried Fruit

Fruits have beautiful shapes, colors, tastes, and textures. Fruits are rich sources of vitamins and are low in fat and calories. Fruits are rich in a wide variety of phytochemicals. These are marvelous compounds that help prevent cancer, prevent free-radical damage to tissues, and are beneficial in so many ways.

Fruits are broadly classified into four groups. *Drupes* are fleshy fruits with a hard pit inside. Peaches, plums, olives, apricots, and cherries are in this group. *Pomes* are fleshy fruit with a thin skin with seeds in the center. Apples and pears are the main examples in this group. *Berries* are a fleshy fruit with many seeds inside. These include blueberries, grapes, cranberries, papaya, and even bananas. *Hesperidia* are fruits with a leathery outside and fleshy fruit inside. Oranges, lemons (considered in chapter 3 on citrus), and cantaloupes are in this group.

The vegan Seventh-day Adventists eat more freely of fresh fruit than the other diet groups.[1]

Figure 1. The daily average consumption of fresh fruit in grams per day by Seventh-day Adventists in five diet categories[2]

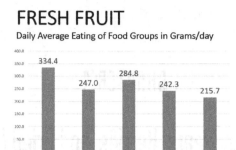

Ellen White felt that apples were a superior fruit.

> If you can get apples, you are in a good condition as far as fruit is concerned, if you have nothing else ... I do not think such large varieties of fruit are essential, yet they should be carefully gathered and preserved in their season for use when there are no apples to be had. Apples are superior to any fruit for a standby that grows.[3]

Ellen White and her family raised and served large amounts of fresh fruit.

> In their season we have grapes in abundance, also prunes and apples, and some cherries, peaches, pears, and olives, which we prepare ourselves. We also grow a large quantity of tomatoes. I never make excuses for the food that is on my table. I do not think God is pleased to have us do so. Our visitors eat as we do, and appear to enjoy our bill of fare.[4]

Berries

There are a profusion of berries, including strawberries, cranberries, blackberries, blueberries, and raspberries, just to name a few. The vegan Seventh-day Adventists eat a lot of berries, as presented in figure 2.

Figure 2. The daily average consumption of berries in grams per day by Seventh-day Adventists in five diet categories[5]

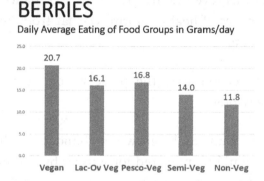

The healthiest Adventists eat almost twice as many berries per day as the non-vegetarian group.

Berries are deeply colored fruit, being dark shades of red, blue, and purple. These intense colors are imparted by a class of phytochemicals known as polyphenols—some known as anthocyanins. There are over eight thousand different polyphenols in the human diet. Flavonoids are another large group (over six thousand) of healthful phytochemicals in the human diet.[6,7]

Berries retard the formation of cancers by several mechanisms[8,9] and have a favorable impact on blood pressure and blood lipid levels that affect cardiovascular diseases.[10,11,12,13,14,15,16] Though many berries are sweet and have a high sugar content, they have a positive effect on blood sugar levels and should be in the diet of diabetics as well as healthy people.[17,18,19,20] It is likely that berries have positive effects on mental function in children, the young, and older adults.[21,22]

Ellen White saw that an abundance of berries was consistent with the principles of a healthful lifestyle.

> Sometimes we gave entertainments, and we took great care that all that we prepared for the table was palatable and nicely served. In fruit season, we would get blueberries and raspberries fresh from the bushes, and strawberries fresh from the vines. We made the table fare an object lesson which showed those present that our diet, even though it was in accordance with the principles of health reform, was far from being a meager one.[23]

Ellen White encouraged the preservation of berries for use throughout the winter.

> Wherever fruit can be grown in abundance, a liberal supply should be prepared for winter, by canning or drying. Small fruits, such as currants, gooseberries, strawberries, raspberries, and blackberries, can be grown to advantage in many places where they are but little used, and their cultivation is neglected.[24]

Dried Fruit

Preserving fruit by drying has been around for thousands of years. Drying fruit removes water, concentrates natural sugars, retards spoilage, and allows for prolonged storage. Dried fruit is mentioned in the Bible.[25]

Drying fruit in the sun is one of the most ancient methods of food preservation. Following simple guidelines, anyone can dry fruit in their own home.[26] While many fruits can be preserved by drying, certain fruits are primarily consumed in their dried state. This includes dates, raisins, prunes, and apricots. The healthiest Seventh-day Adventists eat dried fruit over two and a half times as much as the non-vegetarian group of Adventists.

Figure 3. The daily average consumption of dried fruit in grams per day by Seventh-day Adventists in five diet categories[27]

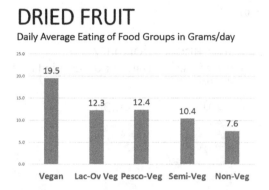

DRIED FRUIT
Daily Average Eating of Food Groups in Grams/day

There are special benefits from eating dried fruit. Among Seventh-day Adventists, the risk of dying from cancer of the pancreas was reduced by over 50 percent for those eating dried fruit even just once or twice a week. There was an amazing reduction of 65 percent for those eating dried fruit three or more times a week.[28]

Figure 4. The risk of dying of cancer of the pancreas for 34,000 Seventh-day Adventists using raisins, dates, and other dried fruit in their diet by frequency of eating in times per week[29]
Significance p = 0.009

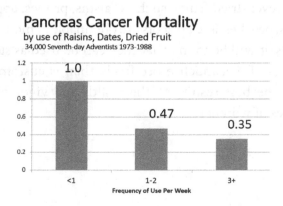

Pancreas Cancer Mortality
by use of Raisins, Dates, Dried Fruit
34,000 Seventh-day Adventists 1973-1988

Frequency of Use Per Week

A similar significant reduction in the risk of developing prostate cancer was found for those eating dried fruit.[30]

Figure 5. The risk of dying of cancer of the prostate for 14,000 Seventh-day Adventist men using raisins, dates, and other dried fruit in their diet by frequency of eating in times per week[31]
Significance p = 0.01

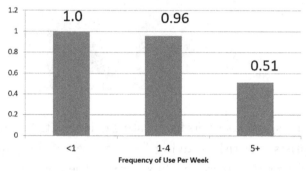

Prostate Cancer Mortality
by the use of Raisins, Dates or other dried fruit.
14,000 Seventh-day Adventist Men

For men eating dried fruit five days a week, the risk of dying of cancer of the prostate was cut in half.

Dried fruit is beneficial to include in the diet. Ellen White encouraged the use of dried fruit in the diet as important for the health and vigor of all.

> Wherever dried fruits, such as raisins, prunes, apples, pears, peaches, and apricots are obtainable at moderate prices, it will be found that they can be used as staple articles of diet much more freely than is customary, with the best results to the health and vigor of all classes of workers.[32]

Eating more apples and berries

Different Ways to Eat More Apples

Baked apples
Apple cobbler
Applesauce
Apples in green salads and coleslaw
Dried apples
Apple tapioca
Apples in fruit salads
Apple butter

Ideas for Increasing Consumption of Fresh Berries

Use berries in a fruit salad.
Use berries in a mixed green salad with toasted pecans.
Use berries over granola or cooked cereal.
Use berries in fruit drinks and smoothies.
Use berries in fruit pies, cobblers, and tarts.
Use berries in jams and preserves.
Use berries over pancakes, French toast, or waffles.

Recipes

Sugarless Apple Pie—serves 6

2 (9-inch) pie crusts, separated
2 tablespoons white flour or Minute Tapioca
1/4 teaspoon cinnamon
sprinkle of nutmeg
1/4 teaspoon salt
6 cups tart apples, sliced thinly
1/2 cup frozen apple juice concentrate, thawed

Place bottom crust in nine-inch pie pan. In a separate bowl, combine flour, cinnamon, nutmeg, and salt. Add mixture to apples and lightly toss with a fork. Place in pie dish and pour apple juice concentrate over the apples. Cover with top crust. Bake 1 hour at 375°F.

Kale and Apple Smoothie—serves 1

1 cup kale leaves, stems removed
1 cup spinach leaves
juice of 1/2 fresh lemon
1 green apple, peeled and cored
1/2 cucumber (optional)
1 teaspoon agave nectar or honey
1/2 cup water
3 ice cubes

Place all ingredients in a blender and blend until smooth. This drink is full of healthy nutrients and is cool and refreshing.

Berry Smoothie (blackberry, raspberry, blueberry, strawberry)—serves 4

2 cups of freshly washed berries
1 cup soy or almond milk
1 cup apple juice
2 tablespoons agave nectar
1 large ripe frozen banana

Place all ingredients in the blender. Blend until smooth. Yield: 1 quart.

Sugarless Berry Jam—serves 8

1 cup fresh berries
1/2 cup dried pineapple
1/2 teaspoon fresh lemon juice

Place all ingredients in blender and blend until almost smooth. This jam should be stored in the refrigerator and used within two weeks.

Berry Topping

1/2 cup water
3 ounces frozen apple juice concentrate or other berry flavors, thawed
1/4 teaspoon vanilla
4 teaspoons cornstarch mixed with ¼ cup water
1 cup berries

Combine all the ingredients except the fresh berries in a saucepan. Bring to a boil. When thickened, remove from heat and add the berries. Gently stir to combine. Serve warm over pancakes or waffles.

CHAPTER 5

Vegetables: Foundation Foods of a Healthy Diet

There are many reasons vegetables should be a major component in the diet. They might not be the most popular foods, but they add color, flavor, and texture to the diet. Vegetables are an excellent source of many nutrients, phytochemicals, and dietary fiber not plentiful in other foods.

Proper preparation, storage, and handling of vegetables are essential to retain these desirable qualities. You can hardly get a well-balanced diet without vegetables.

Vegetables are the roots, tubers, bulbs, stems, leaves, flowers, and seeds of plants. Certain fruits are usually considered vegetables, including tomatoes, squash, pumpkin, melons, peppers, and eggplant. Beans and legumes are also vegetables, but because of their high protein content, they will be addressed in a separate chapter.

Vegetables are the lowest in calories as compared to starchy foods, grains, meats, dairy, and even fruits. They also contain large amounts of fiber, essential to health. Of equal importance to good nutrition are the four main colorful pigments found in plants: red, green, yellow, and white. Each colorful pigment contributes powerful phytochemicals that protect the body against disease.

Ellen White, her family, and her staff planted large gardens and raised a wide variety of fruits and vegetables. She frequently mentions her garden in her correspondence. Here is an excerpt from a letter written when she was living in Cooranbong, New South Wales, Australia.

> Though it was very late last year when our vegetables were planted, and though we had no rain except a few showers from March to October, yet the yield of squashes, melons, peas, beans, cucumbers, carrots, and tomatoes has been excellent. Our orchards also are doing very well. The coming season we hope the crops will do much better. Quite a space of land has been cleared, and the vegetables will be planted earlier. Our second crop of peas is now up, and the potatoes we have planted are up and doing well.[1]

Vegetables can be organized into subgroups: dark-green, starchy, red and orange, beans and peas, and other legumes. Beans and peas will be addressed in the protein chapter. All dietary groups of Seventh-day Adventists eat significant quantities of vegetables.[2] Vegan Seventh-day Adventists eat about 25 percent more vegetables than non-vegetarian Seventh-day Adventists.

Figure 1. The daily average consumption of vegetables in grams per day by Seventh-day Adventists in five diet categories[3]

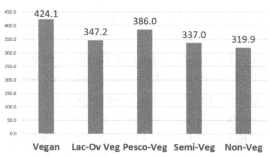

VEGETABLES
Daily Average Eating of Food Groups in Grams/day

An international study including over three hundred thousand participants in eighteen high-, medium-, and low-income countries in North and South America, Europe, the Middle East, Asia, and Africa showed that no matter who you are and no matter where you live, vegetables—even in modest quantities—greatly reduce your risk of dying.[4] Here are the data on all causes of mortality. Having three servings of vegetables a day resulted in a more than a 25 percent reduction in the risk of dying of both cardiovascular causes and cancer.

Figure 2. Risk of dying of any cause for 300,000 men and women (non-Seventh-day Adventists) from around the world by the number of servings of vegetables in their diet per day[5]
Significance p = <0.0001

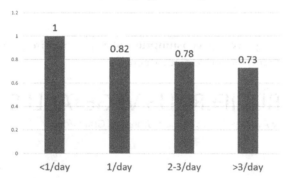

Overall Mortality by Vegetable Intake in Servings per day

Cruciferous Vegetables

One important category of vegetables is cruciferous vegetables. These vegetables include arugula, bok choy, broccoli, brussels sprouts, cabbage, cauliflower, collard greens, horseradish, kale, radishes, rutabaga, turnips, and wasabi.[6]

Cruciferous vegetables are rich in nutrients, including several carotenoids (beta-carotene, lutein, zeaxanthin); vitamins C, E, and K; folate; and several minerals. They also are a good fiber source.

Cruciferous vegetables contain a group of substances known as glucosinolates, which are sulfur-containing chemicals. These chemicals are responsible for the pungent aroma and bitter flavor of cruciferous vegetables.[7]

During food preparation, chewing, and digestion, the glucosinolates in cruciferous vegetables are broken down to form biologically active compounds such as indoles, nitriles, thiocyanates, and isothiocyanates.[8]

These powerful chemical compounds help protect cells from DNA damage, help inactivate carcinogens, and have antiviral, antibacterial, and anti-inflammatory effects. They induce cell death in cancer cells and inhibit blood vessel formation in tumors and cancer cell migration to distant sites in the body.[9]

The cancers in humans prevented by eating cruciferous vegetables include colorectal cancer, prostate cancer, and cancers of the lung and breast.[10] The vegan Seventh-day Adventists eat the most cruciferous vegetables.

Figure 3. The daily average consumption of vegetables in grams per day by Seventh-day Adventists in five diet categories[11]

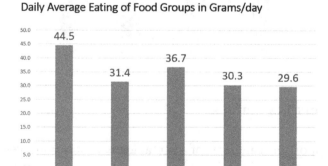

CRUCIFEROUS VEGETABLES
Daily Average Eating of Food Groups in Grams/day

Ellen White obtained greens from multiple cultivated and wild sources.

But as far as material for greens is concerned, you need have no concern; for to my certain knowledge there are in the section of country where you live many kinds of vegetable productions which I can use as greens. I shall be able to obtain the leaves of the yellow dock, the young dandelion, and mustard.[12]

She also enjoyed turnip greens.

The very day I arrived we rode out and gathered nice new turnip greens. We are beginning to get used to Oakland a little now. But it has been raining last night and this forenoon.[13]

Potatoes

Potatoes are not usually considered particularly nutritious. This is a mistake. The food industry insults potatoes by powdering them for instant mashed potatoes, deep fat frying them, or making high-fat, salty chips out of them. Vegan Seventh-day Adventists eat the largest amount of white potatoes, but only about 25 percent more than the non-vegetarian Seventh-day Adventists.[14]

Figure 4. The daily average consumption of white potatoes in grams per day by Seventh-day Adventists in five diet categories[15]

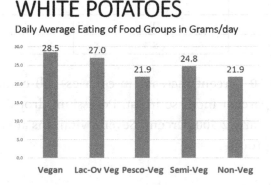

WHITE POTATOES
Daily Average Eating of Food Groups in Grams/day

Vegan: 28.5 | Lac-Ov Veg: 27.0 | Pesco-Veg: 21.9 | Semi-Veg: 24.8 | Non-Veg: 21.9

The opposite is true with fried potatoes. The non-vegetarians prefer French fries more than twice as much as the vegans.[16]

Figure 5. The daily average consumption of fried potatoes in grams per day by Seventh-day Adventists in five diet categories[17]

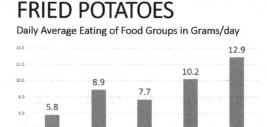

FRIED POTATOES
Daily Average Eating of Food Groups in Grams/day

Some characteristics of potatoes drastically change with deep fat frying. These changes are summarized in this table.

Nutrient Properties of a Baked Potato and French Fries, 100 Gram Portion[18]		
Nutrient	Baked Russet Potato	French Fries Regular Cut, Salted
Water (grams)	74.5	67.1
Calories	97	150
Total Fat (grams)	0.13	5.0
Sodium (mg)	14	349
Potassium (mg)	550	380
Calcium	18	13
Vitamin A (IU)	10	4
Vitamin C (mg)	8.3	7.7

Note the 50 percent increase in calories—all coming from the nearly 4,000 percent increase in fat. Potassium drops while sodium increases by nearly 2,500 percent. Several vitamins are also degraded in the frying process.

Ellen White had reservations about frying potatoes but enjoyed baked and boiled potatoes and sweet potatoes.

> We do not think fried potatoes are healthful, for there is more or less grease or butter used in preparing them. Good baked or boiled potatoes served with cream and a sprinkling of salt are the most healthful. The remnants of Irish and sweet potatoes are prepared with a little cream and salt and rebaked, and not fried; they are excellent.[19]

Sweet potatoes are like white potatoes regarding many nutrients, but sweet potatoes have more sugars (which make them sweet) and more vitamins carried in the yellow and orange pigments. Here is a comparison of a few selected nutrients comparing sweet potatoes with white potatoes.

Nutrient Properties of Sweet Potatoes and White Potatoes, 100 Gram Portion		
Nutrient	Sweet Potato[20]	White Potato[21]
Calories kcal	76	86
Fiber, Dietary (Grams)	2.5	1.8
Sugars, Total (Grams)	5.74	0.89
Calcium (mg)	27	8
Vitamin C (mg)	12.8	7.4
Carotene, beta (µg)	9444	1
Vitamin A (IU)	15,740	2

The vegan and pesco-vegetarian Seventh-day Adventists eat the greater amounts of sweet potatoes.

Figure 6. The daily average consumption of sweet potatoes in grams per day by Seventh-day Adventists in five diet categories[22]

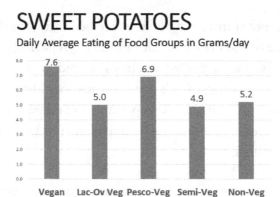

SWEET POTATOES
Daily Average Eating of Food Groups in Grams/day

Vegan 7.6 | Lac-Ov Veg 5.0 | Pesco-Veg 6.9 | Semi-Veg 4.9 | Non-Veg 5.2

Tomatoes

One fruit usually classified as a vegetable is the tomato. Tomatoes are the fourth most popular fresh-market vegetable, behind potatoes, lettuce, and onions. Tomatoes are an excellent source of vitamins A, B6, C, K, E, biotin, folate, and niacin. Tomatoes contain several minerals, including molybdenum, copper, potassium, manganese, and phosphorus.[23] The healthiest Seventh-day Adventists eat more tomatoes than the non-vegetarian Seventh-day Adventists.

Figure 7. The daily average consumption of tomatoes in grams per day by Seventh-day Adventists in five diet categories[24]

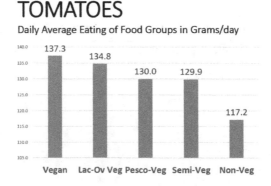

TOMATOES
Daily Average Eating of Food Groups in Grams/day

Vegan 137.3 | Lac-Ov Veg 134.8 | Pesco-Veg 130.0 | Semi-Veg 129.9 | Non-Veg 117.2

Tomatoes were one of the favorite foods of Ellen White. She raised and canned large quantities of tomatoes. Her housekeeper at the time, a Mrs. Nelson, did much of the canning. She mentions this in a letter to her son and daughter-in-law.

> She has already canned one hundred and thirty-eight quarts of tomatoes, sixty quarts of loganberries, and seventy-five quarts of applesauce, besides cherries, peaches, and apricots. We hope to have 200 quarts of tomatoes put up. We have nearly a bushel of sweet corn dried, and have had sweet corn on the table nearly every day for two or three weeks. [25]

At one time tomatoes were a major component of Ellen White's diet.

> I eat the most simple food, prepared in the most simple way. For months my principal diet has been vermicelli and canned tomatoes, cooked together. This I eat with zwieback. Then I have also stewed fruit of some kind and sometimes lemon pie. Dried corn, cooked with milk or a little cream, is another dish that I sometimes use. [26]

There are many health benefits from including tomatoes in the diet. No benefit is more dramatic than the reduction in cancer of the ovary that comes from including tomatoes in the diet regularly. [27] For women consuming tomatoes five or more times a week, there is a 66 percent reduction in the risk of developing ovarian cancer.

Figure 8. Risk of ovarian cancer among 13,000 Seventh-day Adventist women by the amount of tomatoes in their diet[28]
Significance p = 0.002

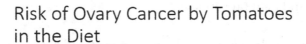

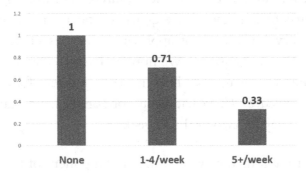

Risk of Ovary Cancer by Tomatoes in the Diet

About 22,200 women are newly diagnosed with ovarian cancer each year. About fourteen thousand women will die from ovarian cancer annually. Ovarian cancer is the fifth most frequent cause of cancer deaths among women, accounting for more deaths than any other cancer of the female reproductive system.[29]

Increasing Vegetables in the Diet

Vegetables can be added to the diet in a variety of ways. They are eaten raw, cooked, or processed. Processing such as canning, freezing, and dehydration makes vegetables more convenient to use and provides them at all seasons of the year. Canned vegetables lose about a third of the water-soluble vitamins as compared to fresh.

Vegetables are a major source of vitamins A and C in the diet, and they also supply some B vitamins and minerals. Vitamin losses in vegetables slowly begins as soon as vegetables are harvested. Nutrient losses continue to occur with lengthy storage, cooking, and processing. For the highest nutrient retention, vegetables should be eaten straight from the garden to the table!

Preparation of Vegetables

Keep in mind that the method of preparation of vegetables is in direct relationship with the retention of color, flavor, texture, and nutrient availability. Listed are a few reminders to keep in mind when preparing vegetables.

1. Vegetables cooked in larger-size pieces retain more nutrients.
2. Cook vegetables only until slightly tender. Overcooking destroys the color, texture, and flavor.
3. Cover the pan while cooking vegetables. Nutrients can be lost in the steam.
4. Use a small amount of water and save it for later soups or sauces. The water contains nutrients leeched out in the cooking process. Liquid from the canned vegetables can also be used in other dishes.
5. Some vegetables can be baked whole in their skins, avoiding the loss of flavor and nutrients.
6. Most fresh vegetables keep best when refrigerated or stored in cool places.

The following recipe makes it easy to consume more vegetables every day—and it is easy to put together. Many variations can be made of this recipe. Be creative and remember that almost anything can be combined in a salad!

One-Dish Salad Bowl

There are five categories of food in the lists below. There are many foods in each category to be combined with foods from each of the remaining categories. Combining at least one or two items from each category can create a whole meal! Vegetables can be cut/torn in bite-size pieces or chopped smaller. The one-dish salad bowl is a good way to use leftovers.

Category One—Cooked Whole Grains

1. Brown rice
2. Quinoa
3. Wild rice
4. Corn
5. Couscous
6. Bulgur/cracked wheat
7. Whole-grain pasta
8. Oat groats
9. Amaranth
10. Barley

Category Two—Raw or Cooked Vegetables
(cut in bite-size pieces)

1. Kale, spinach, chard, bok choy
2. Lettuce, romaine, endive, etc.
3. Asparagus
4. Carrots
5. Broccoli
6. Cauliflower
7. Bell peppers—red, yellow, green
8. Zucchini
9. Green beans
10. Tomatoes
11. Cucumber
12. Brussels sprouts
13. Radishes
14. Onions, shallots
15. Cabbage, red or green

Category Three—Proteins

1. Nuts: walnuts, pecans, almonds, etc.
2. Seeds: sesame, flax, poppy, sunflower
3. Eggs, hard-boiled
4. Beans: black, white, red, etc.
5. Garbanzos
6. Edamame
7. Tofu
8. Lentils
9. Cheese
10. Soy-based meat analogs

Category Four—Seasonings, Sauces*

1. Fresh or dried herbs: oregano, dill, cilantro, thyme, etc.
2. Spices: cumin, garlic, paprika, turmeric, etc.
3. Vinaigrette-type dressings
4. Olive oil
5. Lemon juice
6. Salsa
7. Pesto
8. Tahini

Category Five—Extras

1. Fresh fruit: berries, apple, pineapple, mandarin oranges
2. Dried fruit: raisins, cranberries apricots, cherries
3. Sun-dried tomatoes
4. Olives
5. Capers
6. Avocados

*Note:

Dressings can vary from store brands to homemade.

CHAPTER 6

Salads: The Healthy Way to Go

S alads are an important part of a healthy diet. Greens are rich in vitamins and minerals and are low in calories. Salads are more frequently eaten by the healthiest Seventh-day Adventists. Vegan Adventists eat nearly 40 percent more green leafy vegetables compared with non-vegetarian Adventists.[1]

Figure 1. The daily average consumption of green leafy vegetables in grams per day by Seventh-day Adventists in five diet categories[2]

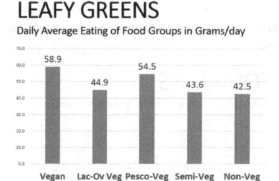

LEAFY GREENS
Daily Average Eating of Food Groups in Grams/day

Eating salads on a regular basis has dramatic benefits, demonstrated in a reduced risk of death as a result.[3] There is a clear dose-response relationship. The more frequently salad is eaten, the lower the chance of dying. A person eating a green salad every day of the week experiences a 33 percent reduction in the chance of dying. There isn't a pill on the market that can reduce the risk of dying of otherwise healthy people more than a fresh green salad every day!

Figure 2. The risk of dying of all causes by the frequency of green salad in the diet of Seventh-day Adventists[4]
Significance p = 0.01

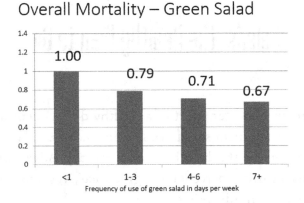

Tomatoes are technically classified as a fruit and are used in a wide variety of ways. For example, they are common ingredient in salads. Tomatoes are relished by the healthiest Seventh-day Adventists.[5]

Figure 3. The daily average intake of tomatoes by Seventh-day Adventists in five diet categories[6]

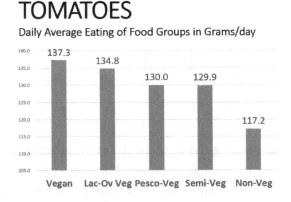

Avocados are unique among fruit. Avocados are a nutrient and phytochemical-dense food moderate in fiber, low in sugar, and rich in many vitamins, minerals, and phytochemicals. Avocados are the only fruit high in fat. Avocado oil consists of 71 percent monounsaturated fatty acids, 13 percent polyunsaturated fatty acids, and only 16 percent saturated fatty acids.[7] This helps to promote healthy blood lipid profiles.

The healthiest Adventists eat the most avocados, consuming nearly three times as much as non-vegetarian Seventh-day Adventists.[8]

Figure 4. The daily average intake of avocados by the five diet categories of Seventh-day Adventists[9]

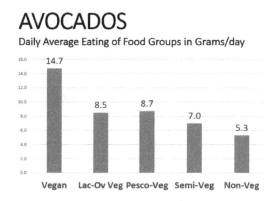

AVOCADOS
Daily Average Eating of Food Groups in Grams/day

CHAPTER 7

Healthy People Go Nuts

A ll nuts grow on trees except peanuts, which belong in the legume family. Nuts are an important component in the diet. Though nuts are high in fat, the fat is largely monounsaturated fat, which is particularly healthful. The protein in nuts is excellent. Seventh-day Adventists eat a lot of nuts. The vegan Adventists eat more than twice as much nuts as the non-vegetarian group.[1]

Figure 1. The daily average consumption of tree nuts by Seventh-day Adventists in five dietary categories[2]

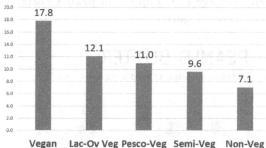

TREE NUTS
Daily Average Eating of Food Groups in Grams/day

Seventh-day Adventists also consume a lot of peanuts, which are widely considered to be nuts but are in the legume family along with peas, beans, and lentils. Though peanuts are a healthful food item, they aren't up to the same quality as tree nuts. Vegan Seventh-day Adventists eat the fewest number of peanuts among the five Adventist food groups.

Figure 2. The daily average peanut consumption of Seventh-day Adventists by five dietary categories[3]

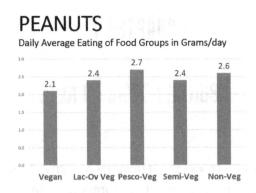

Peanut butter is firmly entrenched in the diet of children and many adults. Peanut butter was not invented by George Washington Carver, as many believe, but by a Seventh-day Adventist physician, Dr. John Harvey Kellogg in 1895. Carver did discover three hundred uses for peanuts, and his innovations increased the legume's popularity and helped make peanuts a staple in the American diet.[4]

Peanut butter has been a popular diet item among Seventh-day Adventists.[5]

Figure 3. The daily average consumption of peanut butter by Seventh-day Adventists in five dietary categories[6]

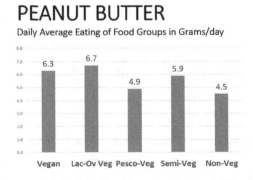

The importance of nuts in the diet gained national attention in 1992 when the staff of the Adventist Health Study published a groundbreaking study showing that nuts dramatically reduced the risk of heart attacks.[7] The study was based on data obtained from the heath records of 31,208 Seventh-day Adventist men and women living in California who were followed for six years. There were 723 deaths from heart disease, and 134 cases of nonfatal heart attacks. A further analysis of these data was published in 1999 with more detail.[8]

Nuts eaten daily resulted in almost a 60 percent reduction in heart attacks. This included men and women, those who were young and old, those who exercised and those who didn't, and those who were vegetarian and those who ate meat regularly. Look at specific subgroups to see where nuts have the most benefit.

Figure 4. The relative risk of experiencing a fatal heart attack by frequency of nut consumption in 34,000 Caucasian California Seventh-day Adventists stratified for age and sex[9]
Significance p = 0.001

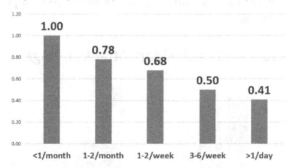

Relative Risk of Fatal Heart Attacks by Frequency of Nut Consumption

Heart disease is the number one cause of death in the United States for both men and women. In this study, nuts benefited both men and women. At the intermediate dose of eating nuts one to four times a week, women appear to have more advantage, but when the full dose of nuts five or more times a week is examined, men have a 60 percent reduction and women have a 49 percent reduction in heart attacks.

Figure 5. The relative risk of a fatal heart attack by nut consumption for men and women[10]
Significance p = <0.001

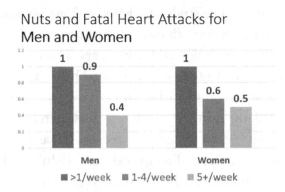

Nuts might be expected to have more benefit for younger people. As a person ages, diseases of several types become more prevalent. It was a significant surprise to find that nuts in the diet were equally protective for both young and old. Notice that even those over the age of eighty had a 55 percent reduction in heart attacks compared with other eighty-year-old people who ate nuts less than once a week.

Figure 6. The relative risk of a fatal heart attack by nut consumption by age.[11]
Significance p = <0.001

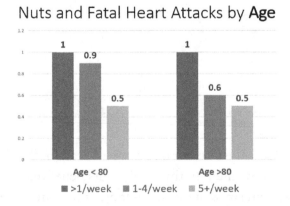

Studies have shown that a vegetarian diet had a moderate benefit in reducing the risk of having a heart attack. In this study, vegetarians experienced a benefit with a lower weekly dose of nuts than non-vegetarians. But at the highest intake of nuts, both vegetarians and non-vegetarians had an equal benefit of almost a 50 percent reduction in heart attacks at the dose of eating nuts five days a week or more.

Figure 7. The relative risk of a fatal heart attack by nut consumption by vegetarian and non-vegetarian diet[12]
Significance p = <0.001 for vegetarians and p = <0.05 for non-vegetarians

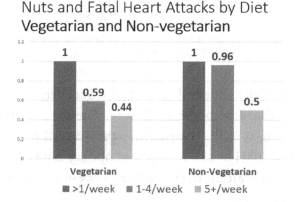

It is well known that exercise has many benefits. Exercise reduces the risk of having heart attacks and helps to control weight, lowers blood pressure, relieves stress, reduces depression, and is important in any healthful lifestyle. In this study, nuts combined with exercise proved to have synergistic effects. Those who exercised less still had a benefit from eating nuts frequently but not as much as the benefit experienced by those who exercised more and ate nuts regularly.

Those with less exercise had a 37 percent reduction in heart attacks by eating nuts, but those who exercised more had a 62 percent reduction in heart attacks by eating nuts five days a week or more. Don't eat nuts while you run or jog as you might choke on them, but combine both for a more healthful life.

Figure 8. The relative risk of a fatal heart attack and nut consumption by exercise level[13]
Significance p = <0.05 for less exercise and p = <0.001 for more exercise

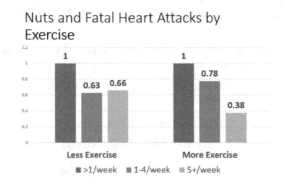

Obesity is a risk factor for heart attacks, but even here, nuts proved protective for those who weighed more. The subjects were divided by BMI (body mass index). Normal weight is a BMI from 18.0 to 24.9. Overweight is a BMI of 25.0 to 29.9, and obesity is a BMI greater than 30. In this analysis, all the overweight and obese were compared with normal-weight people.

Again, nuts are very protective—even for overweight and obese individuals, who experienced a 48 percent reduction in heart attacks. The normal-weight people experienced a 53 percent reduction in heart attacks.

Figure 9. The relative risk of a fatal heart attack and nut consumption by BMI (body mass index), normal weight vs. overweight and obese[14]
Significance p = <0.001 for BMI<24 and p = <0.01 for BMI>24

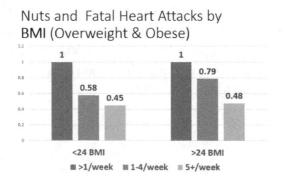

The major risk factors for heart attack include high blood pressure, high cholesterol, and cigarette smoking. In this study, cholesterol levels were not included in the analysis of heart attacks. Cigarette smoking is so low among Seventh-day Adventists that comparisons with the few active Adventist smokers was not practical. Blood pressure, however, was correlated, and here nuts can only slightly blunt the harmful effects of high blood pressure.

Even at high doses, nuts could reduce the risk of heart attacks only by 19 percent in those with high blood pressure. This is still a significant benefit, but it is better to protect your heart by taking blood pressure medication to keep your blood pressure under control. Don't count on nuts to counter the harmful effects of high blood pressure.

Figure 10. The relative risk of a fatal heart attack and nut consumption by blood pressure[15]
Significance p = <0.001 for normal blood pressure and not significant for high blood pressure, p = NS

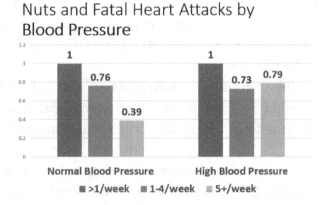

The pressing question at this point is, "What kinds of nuts did these people eat?" Here are the results.

Figure 11. A Table Showing the Types of Nuts Consumed by the Study Population[16]

What Nuts did They Eat?

Type of Nut	Percent
• Peanuts	• 32%
• Almonds	• 29%
• Walnuts	• 16%
• Other	• 23%

Peanuts were the most common nut eaten. Peanuts are not a true nut. Peanuts belong in the legume family with beans, peas, and lentils. The amount and quality of fat in peanuts is good but not quite as good as the fat in tree nuts. As expected in California, where this study was done, almonds and walnuts were the tree nuts most commonly consumed.

The next question is, "How many nuts do you have to eat to get this benefit?" The answer is just a small handful per day. One ounce of nuts equals twenty-eight grams—that is all you need per day. While nuts are high in healthy fats, those who ate this small quantity of nuts every day did not become obese.

The healthiest Seventh-day Adventists eat nuts at least five days a week. It would be a good practice for you to begin. It will reduce your risk of dying from a heart attack and will help you live longer and healthier.

Ellen White recommended the use of nuts and foods made from or containing nuts. Living in California at the time of this writing, she had access to almonds and walnuts and enjoyed both.

> Nuts and nut foods are coming largely into use to take the place of flesh meats. With nuts may be combined grains, fruits, and some roots, to make foods that are healthful and nourishing. Care should be taken, however, not to use too large a proportion of nuts. Those who realize ill effects from the use of nut foods

may find the difficulty removed by attending to this precaution. It should be remembered, too, that some nuts are not so wholesome as others. Almonds are preferable to peanuts, but peanuts in limited quantities, used in connection with grains, are nourishing and digestible.[17]

Subsequent studies of different populations have also shown a cardiac benefit from eating nuts as well. The Department of Nutrition of the Harvard School of Public Health in 1999 reviewed evidence available up to that time regarding nut consumption and the risk of coronary heart disease.[18] The authors reviewed the Adventist Health Study and found similar results from an analysis of the Iowa Women's Health Study of 41,836 postmenopausal women. During five years of follow-up, those eating nuts two to four times a week had a 50 percent reduction in heart attacks compared with women who ate no nuts.

Harvard also reviewed data from the Nurses' Health Study of 121,700 female nurses followed for fourteen years. Here the risk of a fatal heart attack was reduced by 40 percent for those eating nuts five times a week compared to nurses who ate no nuts. This study found that peanuts are not as healthy as tree nuts, and peanut butter has only a slight benefit.

Nuts have many benefits. When you eat at least five portions a week, you can enjoy the full health benefits nuts provide. One study found that people who eat nuts live two to three years longer than those who do not.[19] Most research has been done on walnuts, almonds, and peanuts. However, with more time and research, we will learn more about different varieties of nuts and their individual contribution to the diet.

Fortunately, nuts are found in many parts of the world. There are over seventy different varieties. Most of the common varieties include almonds, walnuts, cashews, pistachios, Brazil nuts, pecans, macadamias, chestnuts, and filberts (hazelnuts).

Individual nuts vary in their own unique combination of nutrients and provide a good source of nutrients such as:

1. Almonds: protein, calcium, and vitamin E
2. Brazil nuts: fiber and selenium (just two brazil nuts a day provide 100 percent of the RDI for selenium for an adult)
3. Cashews: non-heme (plant-based) iron and have a low glycemic index (GI) rating
4. Chestnuts: low GI, fiber, and vitamin C (although much vitamin C is lost during cooking)
5. Hazelnuts: fiber, potassium, folate, and vitamin E
6. Macadamias: highest in monounsaturated fats, thiamin, and manganese
7. Pecans: fiber and antioxidants
8. Pine nuts: vitamin E and high in arginine—an amino acid
9. Pistachios: protein, potassium, plant sterols, and the antioxidant resveratrol
10. Walnuts: alpha linoleic acid, plant omega 3, and antioxidants

There are many ways nuts can be incorporated in our diet. Getting five portions each week is easy. Besides the shelled fresh nuts, there are nut butters and nut milks. Some of the common nut butters are almond butter, peanut butter, cashew butter, tahini (sesame seed butter), and Nutella, which is hazelnut butter mixed with chocolate. Nut milk includes almond milk, cashew milk, and hazelnut milk. These milks and butters are high in nutritional content and have a desirable taste.

The question of how long nuts and nut products can be stored before they go rancid depends on the type of nut. The bad news is nuts can turn rancid because the unsaturated oils oxidize quickly during exposure to light, heat, and air.

The "Eat by date" is different for each nut.[20] At room temperature Almonds stay freshest the longest (9-12 months), followed by Brazil nuts (9 months), and Cashews, Macadamia nuts and Peanuts (6-9 months). Pecans and Walnuts are good for 6 months. Hazel nuts are good for 4 months, Pistachios for 3 months, and Pine nuts only 1-2 months. In the refrigerator most nuts will hold for a year and in the freezer up to two years.

There are reasons why people do not include more nuts in their diet.

1. Nuts are high in calories. Calorie-conscious individuals discard nuts because they feel they are too fattening. One ounce of nuts yields about 170 calories. So, while limited amounts should be eaten, they are packed with many nutrients and, because of the fat content, give satiety to hunger so one does not get hungry as quickly.

2. Nuts are high in fat. Cutting back on fat is important, but other foods by comparison that are also high in fat, such as dairy foods, meats, and processed snack foods, often go by unnoticed.

3. People are unfamiliar with the type of fat found in nuts. Many do not understand that nuts are rich in monounsaturated and polyunsaturated fats, which protect the heart and circulatory system, unlike the saturated fat and cholesterol found in meats and high-fat dairy, which have a harmful effect on the body. The fats found in nuts and seeds contain the omega-3 and the omega-6 fatty acids vital to brain health, boost the immune and cardiovascular systems, reduce severity of dementia and mental decline, and alleviate arthritis and inflammation. The following chart compares the types of fats and carbohydrates found in a few selected nuts.

Figure 12. The Protein, Fat, and Carbohydrate Profile of Selected Nuts in grams.[21] (one ounce portions)

Name	Protein	Total Fat	Saturated Fat	Polyunsaturated Fat	Monounsaturated Fat	Carbohydrate
Almonds	6.0	14	1.1	3.4	8.8	6.1
Walnuts	4.3	18.5	1.7	13.4	2.5	3.9
Pecan	2.6	20.4	1.8	6.1	11.6	3.9
Pistachios	5.8	12.9	1.6	3.9	6.8	7.8

4. Nuts are seen as expensive. Whereas nuts are considered expensive, comparing costs of nuts versus processed snack foods, the price is about the same on a weight basis. The food value found in whole fresh nuts compared with chips or other snack foods is exceedingly higher.

There are many quick and easy ways to include nuts in the diet. Because many nuts come from a tree, they are ready to eat, like fresh fruit. Some nuts are classified as a fruit in the botanical sense, where others are classified as culinary nuts.

Some ways to enjoy nuts are the following.

1. Make your own nut snack mix. Lightly toast almonds and walnuts, with sunflower seeds and pumpkin seeds, in a 160- to 170-degree oven for fifteen to twenty minutes. For extra flavor, toss nuts before baking with a sprinkle of soy sauce and your favorite spices, such as cumin, cinnamon, turmeric, garlic, or other spices. Dried fruit can also be added, if desired.
2. Most nuts, when toasted, make a delicious addition to any green or fruit salad.
3. Chop or slice almonds and walnuts and add them to vegetables or other side dishes such as sweet potatoes, winter squash, or green beans.
4. Pecans and walnuts can be added to muffins, breads, and pancakes. They provide extra flavor and nutrition.
5. Many types of nuts can go into homemade granola. The combination of grains and nuts makes for a complete protein for breakfast.
6. Nuts sprinkled on cooked cereal, such as oatmeal, add protein and flavor.
7. Nuts can replace meat and can provide delicious main dishes, such as loafs, patties, or nut balls.

The best benefit we can get from nuts is by eating them five times per week. The US Food and Drug Administration recommends 1.5

ounces of nuts a day, roughly equal to one-third cup, or about one small handful of fresh nuts. This amount represents an average of eight grams of protein or the equivalent of one ounce of meat in protein content.

Looking at the actual number of nuts in a serving, fourteen shelled walnut halves or twenty-four shelled almonds equal one serving. Other numbers of nuts equal to one serving include sixteen cashews, twenty-eight peanuts, or forty-five pistachios.

In summary, nuts have been proven to be health-promoting, providing not only protection against disease by reducing the risk but by providing valuable nutrients and energy as well for overall nutritional well-being. Nuts are delicious to eat and enhance many dishes when added to them. Nuts have a low glycemic index, so they can be included in diets of people with insulin resistance and diabetes. It has been observed that people who eat nuts eat less junk food. So, keep the nut bowl handy as a reminder to eat nuts every day.

Recipes

Nut Patties—serves 10 (2 patties/serving)

1 cup chopped walnuts or pecans
1 cup cooked brown rice
1 cup whole wheat bread crumbs
1 tablespoon vital wheat gluten flour
1 tablespoon parsley flakes
1 cup finely chopped onions
1/2 teaspoon salt
1 teaspoon soy sauce or Bragg Liquid Aminos or Marmite
1 cup nondairy milk

Combine all the ingredients in a mixing bowl. Use a small scoop or shape into 20 patties. Place on a lightly oiled (or sprayed) baking sheet and bake for 30–35 minutes or until lightly browned. Serve with your favorite gravy.

Oat-Nut Waffles—makes 4 large or 6 small waffles

2 cups quick oats
3 tablespoons sunflower seeds
1 and 1/2 cup nondairy milk
1 teaspoon salt
1/3 cup cornmeal
2 teaspoons vanilla
1/3 cup wheat bran
1 teaspoon maple flavoring
3 tablespoons whole wheat flour
1/4 cup honey or date sugar
1/4 cup pecans or walnuts

Combine all ingredients in a blender and process until smooth and creamy. Let stand to thicken while waffle iron is heating. Place temperature control to low. Blend batter again briefly and pour into a waffle iron sprayed with oil. Bake waffle about 10 minutes or until golden brown.

Nutty Granola—serves 20 (1/2 cup portion)

In a large mixing bowl, combine
5 cups Old Fashioned Quaker Oats (not quick oats)
5 cups of a wide variety of your favorite nuts, broken large or coarsely chopped (pecans, walnuts, almonds—sliced or whole chopped, cashews, sunflower seeds, pumpkin seeds, peanuts, macadamia nuts, etc.)

In a blender, combine
1/2 cup water
1/2 cup oil

1 teaspoon almond extract
1 and 1/2 cups brown sugar
1/2 tablespoon salt
(Optional: add grated coconut or dried fruit)

Mix all ingredients in blender till blended.
Pour over the oats and nuts and stir until all is damp.
Spread thin on a cookie sheet and bake at 200 degrees F, stirring at intervals until mixture is golden brown and dry. This takes 1–2 hours. At higher oven temperatures, the granola will be done sooner but will be a darker brown.

California Walnut Chorizo Meat—serves 10 (1/2 cup portion)

This vegan meat substitute is the perfect complement to a frittata, omelet, burrito, taco, pasta dish, or sandwich. *(Courtesy of the California Walnut Commission.)*

3 cups of walnuts
1 and 1/2 cups of chickpeas, cooked
1 cup of vegetable oil
1 tablespoon white vinegar or lemon juice
1 tablespoon paprika
2 teaspoons salt
2 teaspoons ancho pepper, ground
2 teaspoons oregano, dried
1 teaspoon chipotle, ground (optional)
1 teaspoon cumin, ground
1 teaspoon coriander, ground

Combine all ingredients in a food processor and pulse until walnuts are the size of a grain of rice. Heat if desired, just before use.
Store in refrigerator until ready to use.

CHAPTER 8

Legumes: A Must for Healthy People

R emember the fairy tale of Jack and the beanstalk? According to the story, Jack, a poor peasant boy, made his mother angry by trading their precious cow for a handful of colorful beans. However, even though his mother was infuriated, he did make a very smart nutritional move by trading the cow—a source of high fat, high cholesterol, and high saturated fat beef, and milk—for something much more healthful and nourishing. Beans and other legumes are powerhouses of low-fat, cholesterol-free, nutrient-rich, high-energy foods.

Bean History

Records of beans in the diet date back thousands of years to Bible times. They were included in God's original diet given to man. "And God said, Behold I have given you every herb-bearing seed upon the earth ..." (Genesis 1:29).

In Bible times lentils were used in making flavorful soups and stews. The sons of Isaac began a lifelong feud over a rash transaction negotiated over a pot of lentil stew.

> Now Jacob cooked a stew; and Esau came in from the field, and he was weary. And Esau said to Jacob, "Please feed me with that same red stew, for I am weary."

Therefore his name was called Edom. But Jacob said, "Sell me your birthright as of this day." And Esau said, "Look, I am about to die; so what is this birthright to me?" Then Jacob said, "Swear to me as of this day." So he swore to him, and sold his birthright to Jacob. And Jacob gave Esau bread and *stew of lentils*; then he ate and drank, arose, and went his way. Thus Esau despised his birthright. (Genesis 25:29–34)

Hundreds of years later, King David fled from his son, the traitor Absalom. David and those with him escaped with just the clothes on their backs. A friendly farmer sympathetic to David's cause brought out food and camping supplies for the escaping group. Beans and lentils were part of the feast prepared for David.

Now it happened, when David had come to Mahanaim, that Shobi the son of Nahash from Rabbah of the people of Ammon, Machir the son of Ammiel from Lo Debar, and Barzillai the Gileadite from Rogelim, brought beds and basins, earthen vessels and wheat, barley and flour, parched grain and *beans, lentils* and parched seeds, honey and curds, sheep and cheese of the herd, for David and the people who were with him to eat. For they said, "The people are hungry and weary and thirsty in the wilderness." (2 Samuel 17:27–29)

The most famous reference to beans and lentils in the Bible is found in Ezekiel, where God himself gave the formula for multigrain bread. This is known as Ezekiel's bread and is commercially available today in the freezer section of many health food stores.

Also take for yourself wheat, barley, *beans, lentils,* millet, and spelt; put them into one vessel, and make bread of them for yourself. During the number of days that you lie on your side, three hundred and ninety days, you shall eat it." (Ezekiel 4:9)

This bread formula contains all the nutrients essential for life. Ezekiel ate this bread exclusively for over one year and remained in perfect health.

Reasons to Eat Legumes

1. They are whole foods, not processed, refined, or fractioned foods.
2. They are not secondary foods such as animal food products.
3. They provide essential amino acids in a complete protein when eaten with other grains, nuts, or vegetables.
4. They utilize land space efficiently. It is better for the environment to eat directly from the land.
5. They are economical to purchase and yield high protein per pound.
6. They can be grown in a home garden easily.
7. They provide delicious flavors, pleasing to the appetite.
8. They contain fiber and carbohydrates animal foods do not provide.
9. They are low in fat, cholesterol free, and a great source of vitamins and minerals.
10. They store well, are convenient to use, and are very versatile.

Beans are members of the legume family, which includes a large variety of peas, beans, garbanzos (chickpeas), lentils, favas, and even peanuts. They are characterized by seed-bearing pods that split into two halves. They differ from one another in color, shape, and flavor. Legumes are self-contained packets of proteins, carbohydrates, fats, vitamins, and minerals needed to sustain a sprout until it is big enough to extract nutrients from the soil on its own. Legumes also absorb nitrogen directly from the air, turn elemental nitrogen into nitrogenous compounds that can be used by the plant, and enrich the soil when the plant dies.

Seventh-day Adventists—especially those who are vegetarian—have long promoted beans, peas, and lentils as good replacements for beef, poultry, and fish because of their high protein content. The specific benefits of legumes in the diet were not discovered until the results of the Adventist Health Study uncovered some important information.

The consumption of legumes varies some, as seen in the five dietary groups.[1]

Figure 1. Daily legume consumption of Seventh-day Adventists by five dietary groups.[2]

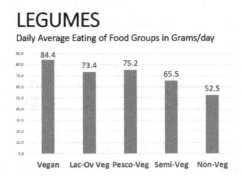

LEGUMES

Daily Average Eating of Food Groups in Grams/day

Legumes Prevent Cancers

Legumes in the diet can greatly reduce the risk of dying from certain cancers. One example is cancer of the colon. Colon cancer is the third most frequently diagnosed cancer in both men and women in the United States, resulting in over fifty thousand deaths each year.[3]

Seventh-day Adventists who ate beans, peas, and lentils regularly had a dramatic reduction in the risk of developing colon cancer.[4] Those who ate legumes once or twice a week had a nearly 30 percent reduction in colon cancer risk, while those who ate beans more than twice a week had a nearly 50 percent reduction in colon cancer. Beans may give you unwanted gas, but they will cut your risk of colon cancer by nearly half.

Figure 2. Colon cancer for 34,000 Seventh-day Adventist men and women followed for five years[5]
Significance p = 0.03

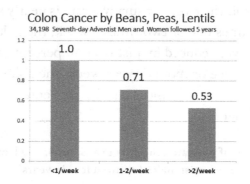

Pancreas cancer is the fourth most common cause of cancer death in both men and women in the United States. There are just over forty thousand deaths from cancer of the pancreas each year.[6]

Seventh-day Adventists who regularly ate beans, peas, or lentils had a significant decrease in pancreas cancer.[7] Even those who ate legumes only once or twice a week had an over 50 percent decrease in deaths from cancer of the pancreas compared with those who rarely or never ate beans. There was even less pancreas cancer among Seventh-day Adventists who ate beans or peas three or more times a week.

Figure 3. Pancreas cancer by beans, peas, and lentils among 34,000 Seventh-day Adventist men and women followed for fifteen years[8]
Significance p = 0.044

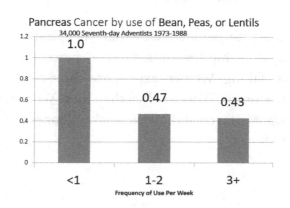

A benefit of equal magnitude was discovered between legumes in the diet and prostate cancer.[9] Prostate cancer is the number one cancer diagnosed in men. Fortunately, with early detection and prompt treatment, the five-year survival rate is nearly 99 percent. For men eating legumes one or two times a week, the risk of developing prostate cancer was reduced by just over 30 percent, while for those eating legumes three or more times a week, the risk was reduced by over 50 percent. Prostate cancer can be prevented by eating more beans, peas, and lentils.

Figure 4. Reduction of prostate cancer by beans, peas, and lentils in the diet in 14,000 Seventh-day Adventist males followed for six years[10]
Significance p = 0.005

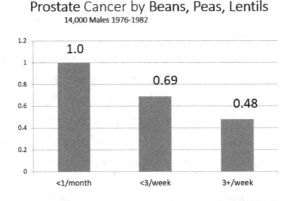

Beans Prevent Hip Fractures

Each year over three hundred thousand people sixty-five and older are hospitalized for hip fractures. Over 95 percent of hip fractures are caused by falling. Women experience three-quarters of all hip fractures, and women fall more often than men. Women are prone to develop osteoporosis, a condition that weakens bones and makes them more likely to break.[11]

Good tests can accurately determine the degree of osteoporosis a person has. Good treatments can reduce bone loss and reduce the risk of hip and other fractures.

The Adventist Health Study examined the role of beans, peas, and lentils in preventing hip fractures.[12] Men and women who ate legumes at least once a week had a 50 percent reduction in hip fractures compared to people who ate legumes less than once a month. Those who ate legumes in some form at least once a day experienced a 64 percent reduction in the risk of hip fracture.

Figure 5. Reduction in hip fractures by beans, peas, and lentils in 33,000 Seventh-day Adventist men and women followed for seven years[13]
Significance p = 0.0003

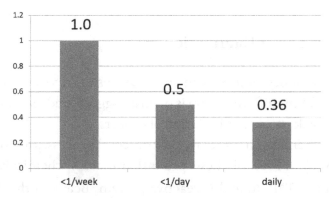

Hip Fractures by Beans, Peas, Lentils
33,208 Seventh-day Adventist Men and Women followed 7 years

Several factors contribute to hip fractures, such as reduced physical activity, decreased muscle strength, low vitamin D levels, and inadequate protein in the diet. Legumes are an excellent source of protein and other essential nutrients. Without specifying the exact mechanism by which legumes preserve bone health, it is enough to say that hip fractures are reduced by eating more beans, peas, and lentils.

Legumes and Cholesterol

Beans have a positive effect on blood fats. Beans in the diet lower cholesterol levels—especially the LDL or bad cholesterol, partially by providing insoluble fiber, which binds to cholesterol and increases its elimination from the body.[14,15,16,17,18]

Figure 6. The effect of beans in the diet on cholesterol levels[19]

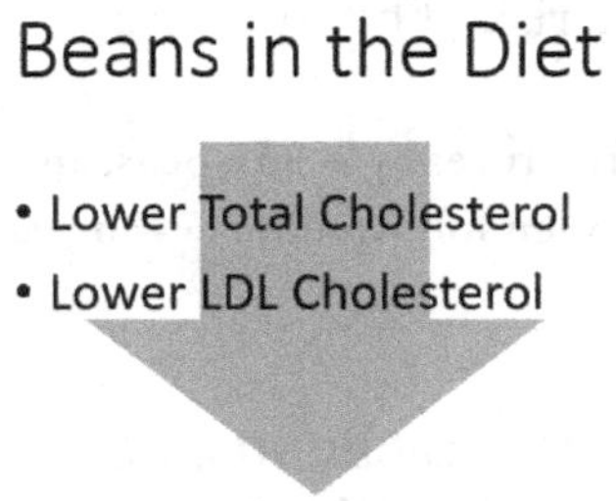

Beans in the Diet

- Lower Total Cholesterol
- Lower LDL Cholesterol

Legumes and Inflammation

Inflammatory processes in the body result in wear and tear on human systems. Inflammation is often a trigger for adverse events like a heart attack, stroke, or initiation of cancers.

Body chemicals indicate that detrimental processes are occurring in the body. Three of these pro-inflammatory chemicals include Interlukin-6, TNF-α, and C-reactive protein. Beans in the diet have been shown to reduce levels of these markers of inflammation.[20]

Figure 7. Beans lower serum markers of inflamation[21]

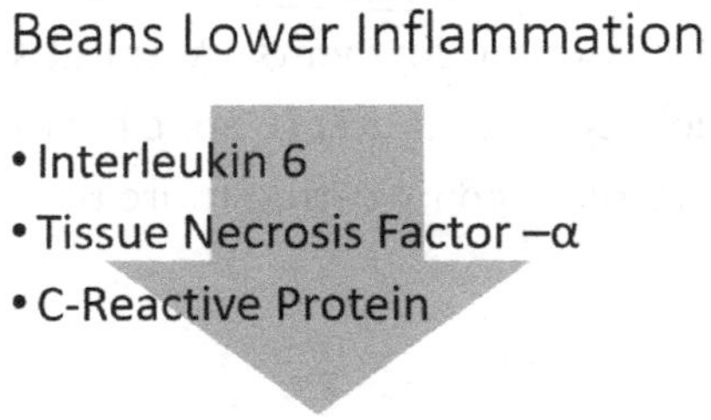

Beans Lower Inflammation

- Interleukin 6
- Tissue Necrosis Factor −α
- C-Reactive Protein

Beans and Appetite Control

Obesity is both a national and global epidemic. Some neurochemical mediators stimulate appetite, while other chemicals help control appetite. Examples of appetite-stimulating hormones go by the cryptic names of PYY, OXM, and ghrelin. Beans in the diet reduce the levels of these hormones. This results in a feeling of satisfaction with the food you eat and prevent overeating and resultant obesity.[22] Beans in the diet result in greater satiety with a smaller meal. Hunger returns later, which curbs snacking between meals. These are important factors in losing weight.

Figure 8. Beans lower neurochemicals that stimulate the appetite.[23]

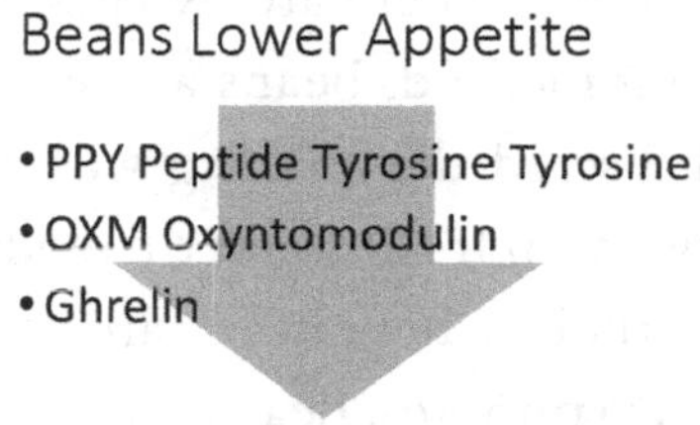

Beans Lower Appetite

- PPY Peptide Tyrosine Tyrosine
- OXM Oxyntomodulin
- Ghrelin

Ellen White recognized the value of beans in the diet and recommended them. She herself could not eat beans, and in her correspondence, she occasionally mentioned her inability to eat legumes.

> Another very simple yet wholesome dish, is beans boiled or baked.[24]

> Some can eat beans and dried peas, but to me this diet is painful. It is like poison. Some have appetites and taste for certain things, and assimilate them well. Others have no appetite for these articles. So one rule cannot be made for everyone.[25]

Recommendations for Cooking Beans

Many people want to eat more legumes but find them difficult to digest. Some of the insoluble fibers can cause gas, bloating, and discomfort. Proper soaking and cooking of legumes can alleviate some of those symptoms. In countries where legumes are eaten as much as three times a day, this does not pose a problem, but where legumes are consumed only a few times a week, they can cause digestive distress in some people.

All legumes need to be sorted to remove dust and any visible debris. Next is a quick rinse before they soak. Soaking reduces the cooking time and improves digestibility. Exceptions to this rule are lentils, split peas, and black-eyed peas, which are thin skinned and may be cooked without soaking. There are two main soaking methods: In the traditional soaking method, beans are soaked overnight; in the morning, drain and discard the soaking water, rinse once or twice more, then boil the beans in fresh water till tender. The other method is a quick soaking method, where beans are covered with water and brought to a boil for two minutes. Beans can stand in the water for one hour, then are drained, rinsed, and cooked in fresh water.

Cooking legumes depend on their age. Older legumes stored for weeks or months take longer to cook than fresher ones. On average beans and garbanzos require two hours of cooking time to be soft and tender. Split peas, black-eyed peas and lentils do not require soaking and can cook in fifteen to thirty minutes. The longer legumes cook the more they fall apart. For soups and stews this is good, but when a whole bean is desired, cook only until tender.

More Cooking Tips

1. Do not add baking soda to beans as it reduces the nutritional value and flavor of beans.
2. Do not add acid food ingredients such as tomatoes, lemon juice, or vinegar until beans are nearly tender.

3. Do not add salt until legumes are nearly tender. Early salting toughens the seed coat.
4. Adding spices too early in the cooking process diminishes their flavor.

Dried legumes can be stored almost indefinitely if placed in a tightly covered container in a dry place. Leftover cooked beans should be covered and stored in the refrigerator up to four or five days. Cooked beans can be frozen in small portions up to six months in airtight bags.

Bean Calculations

1 lb. of dry beans (2 cups) = 6 cups of soaked and cooked beans
1 lb. of lentils (2 and 1/3 cups) = 6 cups cooked lentils
one cup of dry beans serves four people when cooked.

Beano is a commercial preparation proven to lower the incidence of intestinal complaints after eating beans. A few drops mixed with the legumes while cooking is all that is needed. Beano can be found in most grocery stores and pharmacies.

If you would like to incorporate more legumes in your diet, begin gradually by eating one or two portions per week. The 2005 Dietary Guidelines for Americans recommend a weekly intake of six servings (three cups) of legumes per week for people who consume two thousand calories per day.[26] Although legumes are an important part of traditional diets around the world, they are often neglected in typical Western diets.

Bottom line: Legumes are simple to cook, economical, nutritious, and health promoting. They have been shown to lower the risk of many chronic diseases and make for tasty, satisfying eating. There are many reasons legumes should be part of the daily diet, the most important because it just makes good sense!

Recipes

Lentil Roast—serves 6

1 and 1/2 cup cooked lentils (drained)
1 cup soymilk
1/4 cup olive oil
1/2 cup onion, chopped
1/2 cup pecans, as meal, finely chopped or blended whole with soymilk
1 teaspoon garlic powder
1 tablespoon Bragg Aminos or soy sauce
1 and 1/2 cup cornflakes or breadcrumbs

Mix all ingredients and place in an oiled loaf pan or casserole dish. Bake at 350 degrees F for 45 minutes. Serve with brown gravy, ketchup, or BBQ sauce.

Savory Bean Dip—serves 12

1 cup refried beans
1 cup nondairy sour cream
1 cup fresh tomatoes, chopped
14 cup chopped ripe olives
1/4 cup chopped green onions
2 cups nondairy cheddar-type cheese

Mix all ingredients and serve with wedges of pita bread, raw vegetables, baked tortilla chips, or low-fat wheat crackers.

Quick and Easy Three-Can Chili—serves 4

1 (15-ounce) can pinto, red, or kidney beans, undrained
1 (15-ounce) can whole kernel corn, undrained
1 (14-ounce) can tomatoes, diced, whole, or stewed
2–3 teaspoons chili powder

1 teaspoon garlic powder

2 teaspoons onion powder or 1 chopped onion, sautéed

Mix all ingredients and simmer 10 minutes. Serve with wheat crackers or cornbread.

Four-Bean Salad—serves 16

1 (15-ounce) can Great Northern beans, rinsed and drained

1 (15-ounce) can kidney beans, rinsed and drained

1 (16-ounce) can cut green beans, drained

1 (15-ounce) can garbanzos, rinsed and drained

1 pint cherry tomatoes, halved

1 green bell pepper, diced

1/2 cup chopped green onions

1/2 cup sliced ripe olives

Dressing:

1/2 cup lemon juice

3 tablespoons olive oil

1 teaspoon sugar

1 teaspoon dry mustard

1/4 teaspoon cilantro

1 clove garlic, minced

Combine the salad ingredients in a large bowl. Combine the salad dressing ingredients separately in a small bowl. Stir well with a wire whip. Pore over bean mixture and lightly mix to blend. Cover and refrigerate for 1 hour.

CHAPTER 9

Fiber: Nature's Medicine

Dietary fiber is the part of plants not digested when eaten by humans. All plants contain varying degrees of fiber that can't be digested. All meat, poultry, fish, eggs, and dairy products are completely digested and absorbed and do not contain fiber. Refining foods usually removes much of the fiber from the finished product. This includes grains such as wheat and white rice and products made from white flour and pasta.

Since fiber is not digested by humans, it does not contribute to human protein, fat, or carbohydrate nutrition. Nutritionists discounted the importance of food fiber for many years. This was a big mistake. Fiber has a significant impact on human health by reducing the risk of developing several diseases.

Scientists have classified plant fiber into two subdivisions: (1) *insoluble fiber*, which includes cellulose, hemicellulose, and lignin; and (2) *soluble fibers*, which include gums, modified celluloses, mucilages, oligosaccharides, and pectins. Other minor substances not digested include waxes, cutin, and suberin.[1]

The fiber humans can't digest is the primary food source for thousands of different species of microbes in the colon (gut microbiome) that can break down and digest fiber. The health and diversity of the bacteria in the colon have a profound influence on the development of or resistance to several human diseases.[2]

Fiber in grains is rough and coarse. It is found in bran on the outside surface of each kernel of grain. Fiber in fruit is soft and jellylike and is spread uniformly throughout the fruit. Vegetable fiber is found in the walls of each cell of the vegetable, providing shape and stiffness. Cooking vegetables softens the fiber structure, making food easier to chew and swallow.

Fiber expands dramatically in the presence of water and adds bulk to the digestive system. This single fact contributes significantly to digestion. A high fiber diet results in larger and softer stools, resulting in easier bowel movements. The immediate effect is less constipation, less straining at the stool, fewer hemorrhoids, and less diverticulitis and appendicitis. Long-term benefits can include the prevention of IBS (irritable bowel syndrome) and Crohn's disease.

Fiber binds bile salts (which are largely composed of cholesterol) that are secreted by the liver to aid in digestion. In a low fiber diet, after bile salts have helped digest fats, they are reabsorbed back into the bloodstream and used repeatedly. In a high fiber diet, these bile salts are eliminated in the stool, causing the liver to synthesize new bile salts from cholesterol. Therefore, a high fiber diet helps lower blood cholesterol levels, thus reducing the risks associated with hardening of the arteries, heart attacks, and strokes.

Another benefit of a high fiber diet is a reduction in reflux symptoms. This results in a reduction of adenocarcinoma of the esophagus by 33 percent.[3,4]

A high fiber diet results in slower emptying of the stomach contents after a meal. This delays the absorption of sugars and helps control blood sugar in diabetics.

Because fiber adds bulk to the stool, it shortens transit time through the digestive system. This results in favorable effects on human health. The rich and complex society of bacteria that live in the colon thrive on indigestible fiber for their own growth and development.

One such example is certain strains of bacteria that ferment fiber and produce short-chain fatty acids shown to protect against colon cancer, reduce insulin resistance, and raise immunity. One short-chain fatty acid is butyrate, or butyric acid, which helps healthy cells grow and facilitates the destruction of unhealthy cells.[5]

A slow transit time results in prolonged contact of stool with the colon surface before elimination. Bacterial toxins can accumulate, causing harmful chemicals that were complexed in the liver and eliminated in the bile to do damage locally or be reabsorbed to do further damage throughout the body. "Butyrate is recognized for its potential to act on secondary chemoprevention, by slowing tumor growth and activating apoptosis (programed cell death) in colon cancer cells."

A high fiber diet results in a rapid transit time so harmful substances can be quickly eliminated before they can be reabsorbed. The microbiome is altered to more healthful colonies.

There is an industrial marketing push promoting "healthful" bacteria for your colon. These products are called "probiotics." Probiotics contain one to several strains of bacteria thought to be useful in the colon. No probiotic food has the thousands of different species of bacterial colonies found in the colons of healthy people. Most of the bacteria found in the food we eat are destroyed in the digestive process. Then there is the issue of fiber food for these microbes.

Healthful colon bacteria require their own special food. This is the fiber that is indigestible for humans that travels all the way to the colon. Prebiotics are refined fiber products that contain just one or at most a few types of fiber. Inulin is one such fiber sold as a standalone food for colon bacteria.

No commercially prepared prebiotic supplement contains the rich mixture of fiber found in a diet plentiful in fruits, legumes, nuts, and vegetables. To create a supposedly perfect colon environment, a "prebiotic" supplement is combined with a "probiotic" supplement to result in a "synbiotic" supplement. This is designed to induce you to make an unnecessary expenditure on highly refined products containing a few strains of bacteria and refined fiber. All you need is the natural fiber found in ordinary food. This will be more effective than any prebiotic, probiotic, or synbiotic you can buy.

Fortunately, simple changes in the diet can correct your digestive system. Whole grains, fruits, and vegetables have the original, complex fiber needed to result in good colon health. Providing the right environment in your colon will automatically encourage the growth of beneficial bacteria in the colon without having to resort to special foods to manipulate colon fiber or bacteria.

Seventh-day Adventists have long advocated a diet high in fruit, vegetables, and whole grains. The Adventist Health Study has examined these benefits in several studies. Higher amounts of fiber are found in the diet of Seventh-day Adventists. The average US daily fiber intake is fifteen grams. Only the Vegan Seventh-day Adventists do better than the national average. The earliest study of this was performed way back in 1958.[6]

Figure 1. Fiber intake in Seventh-day Adventist men by different diet groups[7]

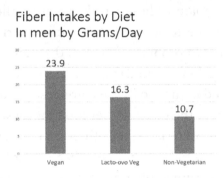

Shown in figure 2 is the daily average weight of the stools produced by different diets. This was an experimental study of fifty-three healthy young adult Seventh-day Adventist males who ate different diets.[8]

Figure 2. Stool weight in young Seventh-day Adventist men by different diet groups[9]
Significance p = 0.05

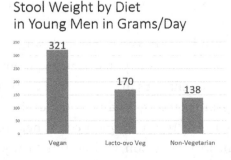

A larger daily stool is an indication of a rich microbiome and residues of indigestible fiber. But does this result in better heath?

Colon polyps are a precursor of cancer of the colon. In a carefully designed study of Seventh-day Adventists, the development of colon polyps was monitored.[10] The study population of 2,818 persons was followed for twenty-six years. During that time, 590 new cases of colon polyps were diagnosed by physicians. The study population was divided into four groups based on the average fiber content in the diet. Those with the greatest amount of fiber in the diet had a 30 percent reduction in developing colon polyps.

Figure 3. Colon polyps in Seventh-day Adventists by the total fiber in the diet[11]
Significance p = 0.04

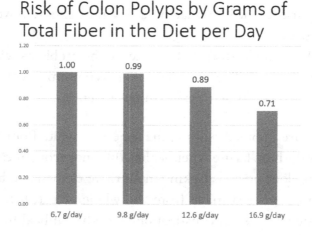

Dietary fiber is not a stand-alone food group. Seventh-day Adventists eat a lot of high fiber foods. Fruits high in fiber include raspberries, apples, pears, bananas, oranges, and strawberries. Grains high in fiber include oatmeal and brown rice. Legumes high in fiber include split peas, lentils, black beans, and lima beans. Nuts high in fiber include almonds, pistachio nuts, and pecans. Vegetables high in fiber include green peas, broccoli, turnip greens, brussels sprouts, and sweet corn.[12]

Ellen White referenced high fiber foods hundreds of times in her writings. In this quote, the first two food categories contain soluble and insoluble fiber.

> Fruits, grains, and vegetables, prepared in a simple way, free from spice and grease of all kinds, make, with milk or cream, the most healthful diet. They impart nourishment to the body, and give a power of endurance and a vigor of intellect that are not produced by a stimulating diet.[13]

A common fiber-free ingredient in most baked goods is refined wheat flour. With losing fiber, there is a loss of vitamins and other phytochemicals. To partially correct the problems with white flour, industry "enriches" it by replacing a few nutrients removed in the refining process.

Ellen White understood before science the problems with highly refined white flour. The most common symptom is constipation, eventually followed by serious vitamin deficiencies.

> For use in breadmaking, the superfine white flour is not the best. Its use is neither healthful nor economical. Fine-flour bread is lacking in nutritive elements to be found in bread made from the whole wheat. It is a frequent cause of constipation and other unhealthful conditions.[14]

The US diet is sadly lacking in fiber. The primary food sources for dietary fiber are the vegetables, fruits, legumes, and nuts that compose a mere 12 percent of the American diet. Processed foods are low in fiber, and many contain no fiber. There is no fiber in meat, dairy, eggs, fish, or seafood.

Figure 4. US food consumption as a percent of calories[15]

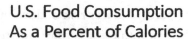

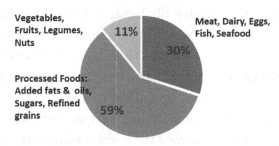

Fiber-containing foods make up only 12 to 14 percent of the foods we eat. Fruits, vegetables, whole grains, beans, and nuts are the only sources of fiber in the diet. Increasing the consumption of these foods in the diet will greatly increase your daily fiber intake. Through figure 4 one can clearly understand why, because of the lack of fiber in the diet, Americans spend an estimated $500 million on laxatives alone, plus the medical costs in treating patients each year.[16]

Most American adults are not eating enough fiber. The average adult only eats sixteen grams of fiber per day.[17] Women need twenty-five grams of fiber per day, and men need thirty grams of fiber per day.[18] Some nutritionists feel this recommended number is still low and that people should probably eat up to forty grams of fiber per day.[19]

Figure 5. Recommended daily intake of fiber for males and females by age[20]

Daily Reference Intake (DRI) of Fiber for Children and Adults		
Ages	Women	Men
1–3	14.0	14.0
4–8	16.8	19.6
9–13	22.4	25.2
14–18	25.2	30.8
19–30	28.0	33.6
31–50	25.2	30.8
51+	22.4	28.0

In a recent study conducted by researchers at the Imperial College in London, those with the highest intake of fiber (over twenty-six grams a day) had an 18 percent lower risk of developing type 2 diabetes than those with the lowest intake (less than nineteen grams a day).[21]

This suggests that dietary fiber may aid people by helping them maintain a healthy weight, which lowers their risk of developing type 2 diabetes. The researchers said that the study only uncovered a "link" between a diet high in fiber and diabetes, and it did not prove cause and effect.

Still, when the researchers focused on specific types of fiber, they found that people who consumed the highest amounts of "cereal fiber" and "vegetable fiber" were 10 percent and 16 percent, respectively, less likely to develop type 2 diabetes than those who consumed the lowest amounts.

An emerging third type of fiber is known as "functional fiber." This fiber is isolated and extracted from whole foods. This highly processed and purified fiber is then added to low fiber foods to "improve" their fiber content. This is not an ideal way to increase fiber intake. Remember "the sum of the parts is not equal to the whole." The way nature packages food is superior to anything industry can do.

In summary, dietary fiber can be soluble or insoluble or both in the same plant. Soluble fiber is found in oatmeal, nuts, beans, apples, and blueberries as examples. It binds with cholesterol, slows the emptying of food from the stomach and absorption of nutrients from the intestines by forming a gel-like matrix, and can add bulk helpful in weight reduction, blood sugar control, and proper bowel functioning. Insoluble fiber is found in seeds, skins of fruit, whole-grain bread, brown rice, and other whole grains. It is beneficial for weight loss, improves GI tract functioning, and can be broken down by helpful bacteria, forming other substances useful to the body.

Figure 6. Fiber content of selected foods. This can serve as a guide in calculating the fiber in your diet.[22]

Fiber Content of Selected Foods		
USDA National Nutrient Database for Standard Reference, Release 27		
Fruits	**Serving Size**	**Total Fiber in Grams**
Raspberries	1 cup	8.0
Pear, with skin	1 medium	5.5
Apple, with skin	1 medium	4.4
Banana	1 medium	3.1
Orange	1 medium	3.1
Strawberries (halves)	1 cup	3.0
Figs, dried	2 medium	1.6
Raisins	1 ounce (60 raisins)	1.0
Grains, Cereal, & Pasta	**Serving Size**	**Total Fiber in Grams**
Spaghetti, whole wheat	1 cup	6.3
Barley, pearled, cooked	1 cup	6.0
Bran flakes	3/4 cup	5.5
Oat bran muffin	1 medium	5.2
Oatmeal, instant	1 cup	4.0
Brown rice cooked	1 cup	3.5
Bread, rye	1 slice	1.9
Bread, whole wheat	1 slice	1.9
Legumes, Nuts, & Seeds	**Serving Size**	**Total Fiber in Grams**
Split peas, boiled	1 cup	16.3
Lentils, boiled	1 cup	15.6
Black beans, boiled	1 cup	15.0
Lima beans, boiled	1 cup	13.2
Baked beans, vegetarian	1 cup	10.4
Almonds	1 ounce (23 nuts)	3.5
Pistachio nuts	1 ounce (49 nuts)	2.9
Pecans	1 ounce (19 halves)	2.7
Vegetables	**Serving Size**	**Total Fiber in Grams**
Artichoke, boiled	1 medium	10.3
Green peas, boiled	1 cup	8.8
Broccoli, boiled	1 cup	5.1
Turnip greens, boiled	1 cup	5.0

Brussels sprouts, boiled	1 cup	4.1
Sweet corn, boiled	1 cup	3.6
Potato, with skin, baked	1 small	2.9
Tomato paste, canned	1/4 cup	2.7
Carrot, raw	1 medium	1.7

Fiber Game: Pick the top ten foods from the table above that are the highest in fiber. List them below. Include them in your diet frequently for good health.

Top Ten Fiber Foods	
1.	6.
2.	7.
3.	8.
4.	9.
5.	10

Recipes

Homemade Black Bean Veggie Burgers[23] —
makes 4 large or 6 small burgers
(13.6 grams of fiber in one veggie burger)

1 can of black beans, drained

1/2 green pepper, diced

1/2 onion

3 cloves of garlic

1 egg

1 tablespoon of chili powder

1 tablespoon of cumin

1 teaspoon of Thai chili sauce or hot sauce (optional)

1/2 cup of whole wheat bread crumbs

1 whole wheat hamburger bun with lettuce, tomato, onion slice, pickles, mayonnaise, etc.

Directions:

1. Preheat oven to 375 degrees F and lightly oil a baking sheet.
2. In a medium bowl, mash black beans with a fork until thick and pasty.
3. In a food processor, finely chop the green pepper, onion, and garlic. Then stir into the mashed beans.
4. In a small bowl, stir together the egg, chili powder, cumin, and chili sauce.
5. Stir the spice mixture into the mashed beans.
6. Mix in the bread crumbs until the mixture is sticky and holds together.
7. Divide mixture into four patties. Form patties with your hands.
8. Place patties on the baking sheet.
9. Bake about 10 minutes on each side.
10. Serve on the hamburger bun with the fixings.

Almond-Honey Power Bar[24]—serves 8
(4 grams of fiber in each bar)

1 cup of Old-Fashioned rolled oats
1/4 cup of slivered almonds
1/4 cup of sunflower seeds
1 tablespoon of flaxseeds, preferably golden
1 tablespoon of sesame seeds
1 cup of unsweetened whole-grain puffed cereal
1/3 cup of currants (or cranberries, cherries, or blueberries)
1/3 cup of chopped dried apricots
1/3 cup of chopped golden raisins
1/4 cup of creamy almond butter (or peanut butter)
1/4 cup of sugar
1/4 cup of honey
1/2 teaspoon of vanilla extract
1/8 teaspoon of salt

Directions:

1. Preheat oven to 350 degrees F.
2. Coat an 8-inch-square pan with cooking spray.
3. Spread oats, almonds, sunflower seeds, flaxseeds, and sesame seeds on a large rimmed baking sheet.
4. Bake until the oats are lightly toasted and the nuts are fragrant.
5. Shake the pan halfway through, about 10 minutes, to mix things up.
6. Transfer the baked items to a large bowl.
7. Add cereal, currants, apricots, and raisins; toss to combine.
8. Combine the almond butter, sugar, honey, vanilla, and salt in a small saucepan.
9. Heat over medium-low setting, stirring frequently until the mixture bubbles lightly (2–5 minutes).
10. Immediately pour the almond butter mixture over the dry ingredients and mix with a spoon or spatula until no dry spots remain.
11. Transfer to the prepared 8-inch-square pan.
12. Lightly coat your hands with cooking spray and press the mixture down firmly to make an even layer (wait until the mixture cools slightly if necessary).
13. Refrigerate until firm (about 30 minutes).
14. Cut into 98 bars.
15. Store in an airtight container at room temperature or in the refrigerator for up to one week or freeze for up to 1 month.
16. Thaw at room temperature.

CHAPTER 10

What to Drink?

Drinking plenty of pure, fresh water every day is vital for your health. Water increases blood circulation. The blood transports nutrients from the digestive system and oxygen from the lungs to every cell in the body. Since our bodies are up to 60 percent water,[1] proper hydration is imperative.

Water from the bloodstream creates urine to eliminate thousands of waste products through the kidneys. Water regulates body temperature, lubricates joints and tendons, and helps maintain the integrity of every cell in the body. Extra water is needed in hot climates and when you are physically active, sick and running a fever, or losing water with perspiration, diarrhea, or vomiting.

There is significant water in the fruits and vegetables we eat. About 20 to 30 percent of our fluid intake comes through the food we eat. The final pathway of carbohydrate metabolism also produces water, which is eliminated through the kidneys, and carbon dioxide, which is eliminated through the lungs. The water produced in this way is termed "metabolic water."

Humans need regular intake of fluids. Besides metabolic water and water from food, we require, at a minimum, the replacement of fluids lost through urination, perspiring, breathing, and in disease states from vomiting and diarrhea. This usually amounts to six to eight 8-ounce glasses of water per day under normal circumstances.

Even more water is needed when there is excessive water loss from exposure to extreme heat or illness. Without concerted effort, most people fall short of this requirement, which places a metabolic strain on the system.

Following is the water consumed by Seventh-day Adventists by the five diet categories. The most water per day is consumed by the vegan Adventists, who drink almost 50 percent more water per day compared to the non-vegetarian Adventists.[2]

Figure 1. The water consumed daily by Seventh-day Adventists by the five diet categories[3]

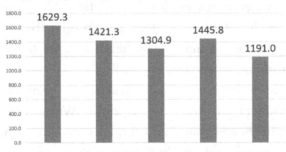

The Adventist Health Study highlighted the importance of drinking adequate water in preventing deaths from heart attacks.[4] These data are based on the experience of over twenty thousand Seventh-day Adventist men and women followed for six years. The risk of a fatal heart attack was reduced by over 50 percent just by drinking five or more glasses of water per day. The data for women was similar and almost reached statistical significance.

Figure 2. Risk of fatal heart attacks for Seventh-day Adventist men by the number of glasses of water drunk per day[5]
Significance p = 0.001

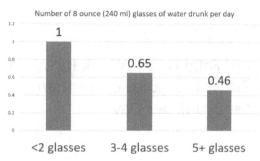

Risk of Fatal Heart Attack for Men by Glasses of Water Drunk per Day

Number of 8 ounce (240 ml) glasses of water drunk per day

Ellen White extolled the use of water in thousands of references. She recommended its use internally and externally.

> In health and in sickness, pure water is one of heaven's choicest blessings. Its proper use promotes health. It is the beverage which God provided to quench the thirst of animals and man. Drunk freely, it helps to supply the necessities of the system and assists nature to resist disease. The external application of water is one of the easiest and most satisfactory ways of regulating the circulation of the blood.[6]

Since all beverages contain mostly water, any drink high in water content might be expected to reduce the risk of fatal heart attacks, but the opposite is true. In this study, the "fluids other than water" category included coffee, hot chocolate, black tea, milk, juices, carbonated sodas, and alcoholic beverages. All these drinks are mostly water.

As the amount of "fluids other than water" increased, the risk of dying from a heart attack increased as well—even though the fluids consumed were mostly water. For Seventh-day Adventist women drinking three to five glasses of "fluids other than water," the risk of dying of a heart attack doubled. For those drinking over five glasses, the risk of dying was almost two and a half times greater than for those who drank less than two glasses of these drinks per day.

Figure 3. The risk of fatal heart attacks for Seventh-day Adventist women by the amount of fluids consumed other than water by the number of glasses drunk per day[7]
Significance p = 0.04

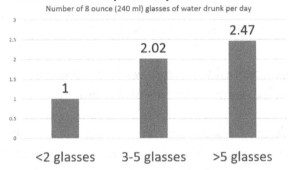

Risk of Fatal Heart Attack for Women by Glasses of Fluids other than Water Drunk per Day

Number of 8 ounce (240 ml) glasses of water drunk per day

This study demonstrates there is no drink better for you than water. As soon as you sweeten, flavor, or otherwise change your drink from pure, clean, clear water, you not only reduce the benefit, but you change something that is intrinsically healthful to a drink that is harmful.

Fluid Intake and Bladder Cancer in Men

Many toxic substances are eliminated from the body through the urine. With increased water intake, toxins are stored in the bladder in a dilute form between episodes of urination. When water intake is low, the kidneys produce a very concentrated urine (with concentrated toxins) as they work hard to maintain hydration by pushing water back into the bloodstream. Concentrated toxin levels in the bladder increase the risk of developing bladder cancer.

An important study of a population of 47,909 health professionals followed for ten years showed a remarkable protective effect of water in preventing bladder cancer in men.[8] During the 435,000 person-years of observation, 252 cases of bladder cancer developed. Cigarette smoking was the strongest cause of bladder cancer.

Water is the most protective fluid to prevent bladder cancer. When other drinks were examined, it was found that coffee, tea, alcoholic beverages, milk, fruit juices, lemonade, and sodas consumed singly or in combination offered no significant protection from bladder cancer. The only protective beverage was water. In this study, drinking six or more cups of water per day resulted in a 50 percent reduction in the risk of developing bladder cancer compared with those who drank only one cup of water per day.

Figure 4. The risk of developing bladder cancer in men (not Seventh-day Adventists) by the water consumed per day[9]
Significance p = 0.001

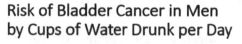

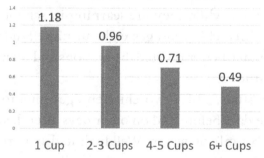

Water in Weight Management

Diet drinks are promoted to help people lose weight. An interesting study looked at water versus diet drinks in helping people to lose weight.[10] This experiment involved sixty-two participants in Great Britain and was not a part of the Adventist Health Study. All were placed on calorie restrictions and increased exercise. Half were instructed to have eight ounces of water after lunch, and the other half were give a diet beverage to drink after lunch. The program continued for twenty-four weeks.

At the end of the study, the water-drinking group had lost 19.4 pounds, while the diet beverage group only lost 16.8 pounds. The difference was statistically significant. Water after the main meal is better than a diet drink.

Another study looking at the effects of drinking water on weight loss was conducted in Birmingham, England.[11] In this study of eighty-four participants, one group was instructed to drink sixteen ounces of water thirty minutes before the main meal, and the control group was asked to simply visualize a full stomach before they ate. At the end of twelve weeks, the water-drinking group had lost almost three pounds more than the group not drinking the water before meals.

Water and Brain Function in Children

Encouraging children to drink plenty of water will help their brains work better while they are learning in school.[12] This study enrolled sixty-three children ages eight to nine. Students with the higher water intake better resisted distractions and maintained better focus in their studies.

In another study,[13] fifty-two children ages nine to twelve were tested on some days before and on other days after drinking twenty-five ounces (750 ml) of water. Well-hydrated children performed several tasks (digit-span task and pair-cancellation task) better than children not encouraged to drink water, thus indicating that water enhances thinking processes in children.

Recommended Times to Drink Water

1. Drink two glasses of water after waking up—helps activate internal organs.
2. Drink one glass of water thirty minutes before meals—helps digestion.
3. Drink one glass of water before taking a bath—helps lower blood pressure.
4. Drink one glass of water before sleeping—may help avoid a stroke or heart attack.
5. Drink a glass of water before and after a workout to replace fluids lost in perspiration and urination.
6. Drink water when tired—fatigue is an early sign of dehydration.
7. Drink water when exposed to germs—it washes away germs and viruses.
8. Drink plenty of water when you are ill. Water helps reduce fever and replaces the fluids lost in respiration, vomiting, or diarrhea.
9. Drink water when you are hungry—it helps take the edge off hunger.
10. Drink water to prevent heatstroke in hot weather. Drink water in cold temperatures to help prevent frostbite.

Sources and Types of Drinking Water

Mountain stream or river water. This water may be crystal clear and cool but usually contains pathogens from wild animal waste. Parasitic infection with Giardia lamblia is a common complication. Surface water should always be treated before drinking it.

Municipal water. Most city water is purified surface water from lakes or rivers. Small-town water supplies may come from wells or natural springs, in which case, significant treatment may not be necessary. Water that comes out of your faucet is most often treated with ozone and chlorine to kill germs and viruses. City water is also filtered through sand beds to remove particulate matter. Strict guidelines are observed, and daily analysis and cultures are obtained to document purity and safety.

Well water. Well water comes from a hole drilled into the ground that taps into an underground water source. Usually, a pump brings water to the surface. Water from wells that pump water through a closed system directly to your house, avoiding contamination from rain runoff, doesn't require treatment and is usually a good source of trace minerals. If you have a private well, it is advisable to periodically have the water tested for minerals, various chemicals, and bacterial contamination. Water from open wells serviced by ropes and buckets is contaminated and should not be drunk without additional treatment.

Distilled water. This water has been turned into steam by applying heat and then condensed on a cool surface. All minerals are removed in this process, and all germs and viruses are killed. Distilled water is recommended as the preferred drinking water for persons with advanced heart failure. It is not a beverage of choice for healthy people since it is devoid of trace minerals and requires tremendous energy to produce.

Reverse osmosis. This water has been forced under high pressure through semipermeable membranes. This removes all minerals and contaminants. This process is ideal for converting salty ocean water into drinking water. Small home-based units are available and may be the treatment of choice for purifying river water downstream from large cities.

Deionized water. This water has all positively and negatively charged chemical ions removed. Deionization is a chemical process that uses specially manufactured ion-exchange resins, which exchange hydrogen and hydroxide ions for dissolved minerals, and then recombine them to form water. Because most nonparticulate water impurities are dissolved salts, deionization produces a high purity water generally like distilled water. Deionization does not remove uncharged organic molecules, viruses, or bacteria.

Artesian or spring water. Spring water comes up through the ground. The water often originates as surface water many miles away and is filtered and purified by traveling long distances through the ground. If the spring is protected from contamination, the water is fresh and contains trace minerals.

Bottled water. This water is sold in plastic bottles and may come from a natural spring or from treated municipal water sources. Though this is convenient, bottled water is more expensive than just drinking a glass of water from the faucet and not any better for you. Bottled water may contain chemicals leached out of the plastic the bottles are made of.

pH-adjusted water. Pure water has a neutral pH of 7.0. The pH scale indicates whether a liquid is more acidic (pH below 7.0) or alkaline (pH above 7.0). Tap water has some slight natural variation in pH depending on its mineral content. Most bottled waters are slightly acidic, and sodas and juices are even more so.

Alkaline water has a pH between 8 and 10. Some are from springs or artesian wells and are naturally alkaline because of dissolved minerals. Others are made with an ionizing process, and water ionizing machines are also marketed for home use.

Alkaline water companies make vague claims it will "energize" and "detoxify" the body and lead to "superior hydration." And some claim that ionized water can prevent everything from headaches to cancer. But there's no evidence that drinking water with a higher pH can change the pH of your body or even that this outcome would provide benefits.[14] As there is no evidence to support the health benefits of alkaline water, there is no recommended amount that improves health.[15]

Many more adjustments to plain water are promoted and sold. Each has some supposed health benefit. Examples include raw water, sparkling water, mineral water, protein water, oxygen water, electrolyte water, fat water, and the list goes on. Nothing beats treated water from your tap.

Filters

There are a variety of filtering systems you can use at home. There are filters installed under a sink providing quantities of filtered water as needed. There are simple pitcher filters that "purify" a quart or two of tap water at a time.

These filters typically remove only a few potentially offending minerals (and sometimes useful minerals), particulate material, or chemicals from drinking water. They rarely represent the highest level of water purification but may be attractive to use if the taste of municipal water is improved with their use.

Biblical References to Spiritual Water

As water is essential for life, just so is Jesus essential for life—eternal life. This spiritual connection with water is so fundamental and profound that Jesus himself made the comparison.

> On the last day, that great day of the feast, Jesus stood and cried out, saying, "If anyone thirsts, let him come to Me and drink. He who believes in Me, as the Scripture has said, out of his heart will flow rivers of living water." (John 7:37–38)

> And He said to me, "It is done! I am the Alpha and the Omega, the Beginning and the End. I will give of the fountain of the water of life freely to him who thirsts. (Revelation 21:6)

Drink water and live. Drink the water of life that Jesus provides and live forever.

Juices

Fruit and vegetable juices are largely composed of water and are extracted from fruits and vegetables. Juices are considered healthful beverages by many people. Popular fruit juices include orange, apple, grape, cranberry, grapefruit, pineapple, prune, pomegranate, papaya, guava, lemonade, and limeade. There are a variety of vegetable juices. They are often combined into a drink and may include juices from tomatoes, carrots, celery, cucumbers, spinach, beets, turnips, or wheatgrass.

Among Seventh-day Adventists, there is fairly uniform consumption of juices across all diet types. The largest fruit and vegetable juices are drunk by the pesco-vegetarians, with the least amount consumed by the vegan Seventh-day Adventists.[16]

Figure 5. The daily average consumption of fruit juices in the five Seventh-day Adventist dietary groups[17]

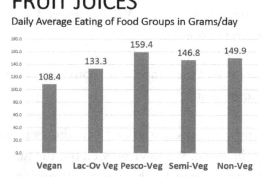

FRUIT JUICES
Daily Average Eating of Food Groups in Grams/day

Fruit juices do not contain the complete nutritional value of the whole fruit from which they were squeezed. The whole fruit contains dietary fiber and is digested and metabolized more slowly than juices. The released sugar in juices enters the bloodstream rapidly and has adverse effects on blood sugar and triglyceride levels.

Drinking fruit and vegetable juices increases sugar and other additives you would not get from eating the fruit or vegetable in its natural state. Consider carrot juice. Often the juice from a dozen carrots produces just one glass of carrot juice. Hardly would one eat a dozen carrots at one setting, but one can easily drink the juice from a dozen carrots in just a few gulps. This increases not just sugar but the calorie content of the diet considerably.

One complication of regularly drinking quantities of carrot juice is the accumulation of excessive carotene compounds in the skin, resulting in a yellowish/orange tint to the skin. This can be mistaken for jaundice, which results from acute or chronic liver disease. Looking at the white of the eyes helps differentiate between these conditions. In the yellow jaundice of liver disease, the white of the eyes becomes yellow as does the skin. In the hypercarotenemia of carrot juice drinkers, the white of the eyes remains white while the skin is jaundiced.

Some juicing machines process whole fruits and vegetables, leaving suspended in the juice pulverized fiber. Juice prepared in this way is preferable to clear juices with no fiber content, which results in a spiking of blood sugar.

Among the fruit juices Ellen White enjoyed were juices from grapes, oranges, and lemons.

> The pure juice of the grape, free from fermentation, is a wholesome drink.[18]

> We are now expressing juice from the oranges and canning the same. We have pressed out the juice from the lemons also, in order that we may furnish palatable drink for hot weather.[19]

Juice Drinks/Beverages

There are many commercial fruit and vegetable drinks. These drinks often contain as little as 10 percent actual juice and are mostly colored, sugar-sweetened water. These drinks have little nutritional value and should not be included in a healthful diet. Read the labels carefully on juices and purchase only those drinks that contain 100 percent juice. Many juices contain a mixture of fruit or vegetable juices and may only contain a little of the juice you are trying to purchase. Often apple or white grape juice is the predominant juice in the drink, contrary to what is suggested on the label.

Carbonated Beverages

Coca-Cola, Pepsi-Cola, Mountain Dew, Mellow Yellow, Dr Pepper, Pibb Xtra, Sprite, Sierra Mist, 7Up, Fanta, Crush, Sunkist, and diet versions of these drinks are some of the most commonly sold carbonated beverages in the United States. In 2018 almost $200 billion was spent on soft drinks in the United States. This industry has about a $5 billion increase in sales each year.

A detailed analysis of carbonated beverages estimates that worldwide 184,000 premature deaths are attributable to these drinks per year. Of this number, there were 133,000 deaths due to diabetes, 45,000 due to heart attacks and strokes, and 6,450 due to cancer.[20] Approximately 25,000 of these premature deaths occurred in the United States.

Soft drinks are primarily carbonated sugar water and artificial flavoring. Most contain significant amounts of caffeine. Phosphoric acid, which soft drinks contain, damages both bones and teeth.

The healthiest Seventh-day Adventists consume only 7 percent of carbonated soda drinks as compared to non-vegetarian Seventh-day Adventists.[21]

Figure 6. The daily consumption of carbonated soda drinks in Seventh-day Adventists by the five dietary groups[22]

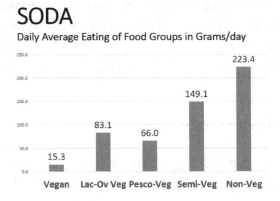

Caffeine Beverages

Coffee, tea, and energy drinks are primarily fluids that dispense caffeine. These beverages are consumed worldwide. US annual consumption of coffee totals over twenty-five million bags of coffee beans, each weighing 132 pounds[23] (60kg), and the United States imports 470 million pounds of tea each year.[24] US sales of energy drinks amounted to approximately 2.98 billion US dollars in 2017.[25]

Coffee

The healthiest vegan Seventh-day Adventists consume a minimal amount of coffee.

Figure 7. The daily average of coffee consumption in Seventh-day Adventists by the five dietary groups[26]

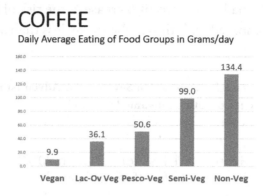

COFFEE
Daily Average Eating of Food Groups in Grams/day

Studies looking for harmful effects of coffee drinking in the general population have produced generally negative results.[27] Coffee drinking by Seventh-day Adventists, however, shows significant harmful effects.[28] A study was done of over nine thousand Seventh-day Adventist men followed for twenty-five years. The harmful effects of coffee drinking were most pronounced for heart attacks—particularly in younger-aged Seventh-day Adventists.

The risk of dying of a heart attack for Adventist men fifty to fifty-nine years of age drinking three or more cups of coffee increased by 170 percent compared with Seventh-day Adventist men who didn't drink coffee or who averaged less than one cup per day.

Figure 8. The relative risk of a fatal heart attack for Seventh-day Adventist men ages 50–59 by the average number of cups of coffee consumed per day[29]
Significance p = <0.001

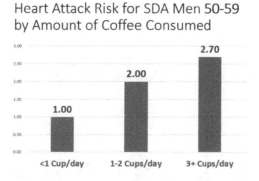

Heart Attack Risk for SDA Men 50-59
by Amount of Coffee Consumed

The numbers were similar for Seventh-day Adventist men seventy to seventy-nine years of age. Here men drinking three or more cups of coffee per day had a 130 percent increase in the risk of having a fatal heart attack compared with those who drank less than a cup of coffee per day.

Figure 9. Risk of a fatal heart attack in Seventh-day Adventist men ages 70–79 by the number of cups of coffee consumed per day[30]
Significance p = <0.001

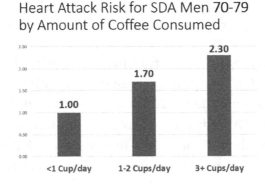

Heart Attack Risk for SDA Men 70-79 by Amount of Coffee Consumed

A better measure of the harmful effects of coffee drinking is on life expectancy or all causes of mortality combined. The risk of dying of any cause for Seventh-day Adventist men ages sixty- to sixty-nine drinking three cups of coffee per day was twice that of Adventist men drinking less than one cup per day. That is double the risk of dying associated with drinking three or more cups of coffee per day. Coffee drinking is clearly bad for Seventh-day Adventists.

Figure 10. The risk of dying from all causes combined for Seventh-day Adventist men 60–69 years of age by the number of cups of coffee consumed per day[31] Significance p = <0.001

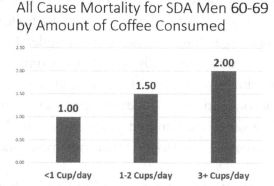

Why should coffee drinking have slightly positive benefits for the general population but have negative effects on Seventh-day Adventists? A clue is found in the decreasing harmfulness of coffee drinking for Seventh-day Adventists as they age. Coffee drinking appears to be less dangerous for Seventh-day Adventists the older they get.

Figure 11. Relative risk of dying of all causes for Seventh-day Adventists drinking three cups of coffee per day by decade of life compared with Seventh-day Adventists drinking less than one cup of coffee per day[32] Significance p = <0.001

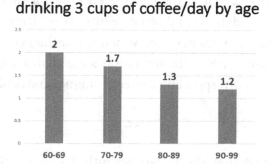

One possible reason for this paradox is that Seventh-day Adventists are so much healthier than the general population. At younger ages,

Seventh-day Adventists are more susceptible to the harmful effects of coffee. Once you look at the effects of coffee on a secular population that adds red meat to the diet and alcohol and cigarette smoking to the lifestyle, and becomes obese, the harmful effects of coffee drinking are lost in the sickness and death that come from a toxic way of life.

As all people age, life becomes more fragile. People acquire the diseases that will eventually kill them. Compared with the accumulation of life-threatening risk factors and diseases, the relative contribution of coffee to the risk of dying appears to diminish.

Ellen White over one hundred years ago advised Seventh-day Adventists not to consume coffee or similar caffeine-containing drinks.

> The action of *coffee* and many other *popular drinks* is similar. The first effect is exhilarating. The nerves of the stomach are excited; these convey irritation to the brain, and this in turn is aroused to impart increased action to the heart and short-lived energy to the entire system. Fatigue is forgotten; the strength seems to be increased. The intellect is aroused, the imagination becomes more vivid.
>
> Because of these results, many suppose that their tea or coffee is doing them great good. But this is a mistake. Tea and coffee do not nourish the system. Their effect is produced before there has been time for digestion and assimilation, and what seems to be strength is only nervous excitement. When the influence of the stimulant is gone, the unnatural force abates, and the result is a corresponding degree of languor and debility.[33]

Tea

It is believed that the vegan Seventh-day Adventists consume primarily noncaffeinated herbal teas. They avoid caffeine drinks, and this influences their selection of teas.

Figure 12. Tea consumption by Seventh-day Adventists in the five dietary groups[34]

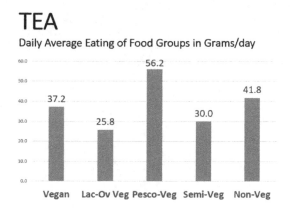

TEA
Daily Average Eating of Food Groups in Grams/day

	Vegan	Lac-Ov Veg	Pesco-Veg	Semi-Veg	Non-Veg
	37.2	25.8	56.2	30.0	41.8

Energy Drinks

Energy drinks, not to be confused with sports drinks, are an increasingly popular source of caffeine. Sales of these drinks exceeded $10 billion in 2018. The top manufacturers are Red Bull, Monster Energy, Rockstar, High Performance Beverage, and Bang (made by Vital Pharmaceuticals, Inc.). The amount of caffeine varies widely in these drinks.[35] Five-Hour Energy Extra Strength contains 240 mg of caffeine in 1.9 ounces of fluid. The average 8 oz. cup of coffee contains from 50-134 mg of caffeine.[36] These are drug-delivering drinks. They should not be included in a healthful diet.

Conclusion

The best beverage is pure water. For the best of health, eat fruit and limit fruit juices. Skip sugary drinks, sodas, coffee, tea (unless it is from herbal sources), and energy drinks.

CHAPTER 11

The Dairy Dilemma

D airy products include milk, cream, yogurt, cottage cheese, sour cream, fresh cheeses, and aged cheeses. We include a discussion of eggs in this section as well. Humans are the only species of mammals that continue to use milk and milk-derived products beyond the first year of life.

Dairy products are characterized as being excellent sources of protein and calcium. The content of butter fat is reduced in many dairy products to lower calorie content and to reduce objectionable saturated fat and cholesterol in the diet.

Milk is the most perfectly balanced food for newborn infants. Babies need nothing more than mothers' nutritious milk. Milk contains proteins essential for growth of muscles and all other living tissues. Milk contains calcium necessary for bone development. Milk contains some of mothers' antibodies to help babies fight off infection until their own immune system can mature. For mothers who can't breastfeed or who opt out of breastfeeding, there are infant formulas that provide balanced nutrition for newborns based on milk or soy.

While milk is provided frequently for children, is milk an ideal food for adults? The Adventist Health Studies have looked at milk intake and correlations with cancer at several sites. While no statistically significant associations with milk and any type of cancer have been identified in these studies, other research has been more conclusive and will be mentioned in this chapter.

When a child is weaned from mothers' milk, cow's milk is introduced. Milk is pasteurized to prevent transmission of infections. There have been concerns expressed about potential adverse effects of milk on growing children. Allergy to cow's-milk proteins is usually transient. Atopic children may independently be at risk for poor growth, and the contribution of dairy nutrients to their diet should be considered.

The connection of cow's milk to autistic spectrum disorder is lacking, and even a cause-effect relation with type 1 diabetes mellitus has not been established because many factors may concur. Although it is true that cow's milk stimulates insulin-like growth factor-1 and may affect linear growth, association with chronic degenerative, noncommunicable diseases has not been established.[1]

All the dietary categories of Seventh-day Adventists use dairy products except for the vegans. There are significant variations in total dairy product use among the other four Seventh-day Adventist diet categories. The pesco-vegetarians and the lacto-ovo vegetarians consume a bit more than half as much as the non-vegetarian Seventh-day Adventists.[2]

Figure 1. Dairy product consumption by Seventh-day Adventists by the five diet category groups[3]

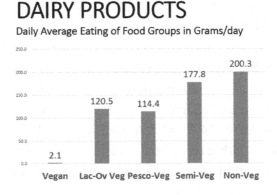

DAIRY PRODUCTS
Daily Average Eating of Food Groups in Grams/day

Milk

Full-fat milk products (4 percent butter fat) include whole milk, cottage cheese, sour cream, and all other dairy products made from whole milk. The lacto-ovo vegetarians and pesco-vegetarians consume less than half that of the non-vegetarian Seventh-day Adventists.[4]

Figure 2. Whole milk and whole milk product consumption of Seventh-day Adventists by the five diet category groups[5]

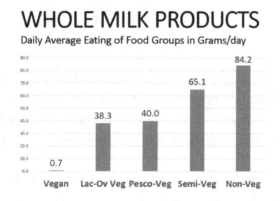

WHOLE MILK PRODUCTS
Daily Average Eating of Food Groups in Grams/day

Low-fat dairy products include low-fat milk, low-fat cottage cheese, and all dairy products made from low-fat milk. The four groups of Seventh-day Adventists that use dairy products use slightly more low-fat (1 percent to 2 percent) milk and milk products than whole milk products. Even more milk products are used by the two groups that include red meat and poultry in their diet.[6]

Figure 3. Low-fat milk and low-fat milk product consumption of Seventh-day Adventists by the five diet category groups[7]

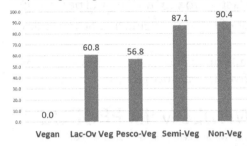

LOW-FAT MILK PRODUCTS
Daily Average Eating of Food Groups in Grams/day

There is no official position of the Seventh-day Adventist church regarding milk and dairy products; its use has been one of individual preference and tolerance. Ellen White correctly observed that many can use milk without difficulty while others cannot use milk at all.

> There is real common sense in health reform. People cannot all eat the same things. Some articles of food that are wholesome and palatable to one person, may be hurtful to another. Some cannot use milk, while others can subsist upon it. For some, dried beans and peas are wholesome, while others cannot digest them. Some stomachs have become so sensitive that they cannot make use of the coarser kind of graham flour. So, it is impossible to make an unvarying rule by which to regulate every one's dietetic habits.[8]

The problem some people have with milk and other dairy products is often due to a lactase deficiency, which was not understood one hundred years ago. The disturbing symptoms of lactase deficiency can be avoided by using milk in which the disaccharide (double sugar) lactose has been broken down into its monosaccharide (single) sugars. Lactaid, a more digestible milk, is available in most grocery stores. Also, over-the-counter pills containing lactase can be taken with dairy products to avoid the annoying symptoms of gas, bloating, cramps, and diarrhea that characterize common milk intolerance.

Raw milk contains infectious bacteria that can cause significant human disease or even death.[9] Even before the days of pasteurization, Seventh-day Adventists advocated heat-treated milk to eliminate the possibility of transmitting disease-causing organisms.

> If milk is used, it should be thoroughly sterilized; with this precaution, there is less danger of contracting disease from its use.[10]

Mrs. White was clear that in her day there was no need to discard milk from the diet if it was properly treated and stored. However, she also added:

> The time may come when it will not be safe to use milk. But if the cows are healthy and the milk thoroughly cooked, there is no necessity of creating a time of trouble beforehand.[11]

Milk, therefore, has been looked upon with some suspicion by many Seventh-day Adventists. Because of these words of caution and other scientific recommendations that have been brought to light by recent research, people today are questioning the safety and hygiene of milk.

> The time will come when we may have to discard some of the articles of diet we now use, such as milk and cream and eggs; but it is not necessary to bring upon ourselves perplexity by premature and extreme restrictions. Wait until the circumstances demand it and the Lord prepares the way for it.[12]

The wisdom in this counsel that was written more than one hundred years ago is that circumstances may demand that milk and dairy products be eliminated from the diet. These circumstances might come from frequent and gross contamination of milk by bacteria or adulterating products. They might also come from definitive information about the harmful effects of milk provided by credible scientific studies.

One study that implicates milk as a cause of cancer, heart disease, and hip fractures was published in the *British Medical Journal* in 2014.[13] This study was conducted in Sweden and enrolled sixty-one thousand women and fifty-four thousand men and followed these people for twenty-two years. This amounts to 1.2 million person-years of observation.

During the study, there were a total of 15,541 deaths among women. There were 5,278 deaths from heart disease and 3,282 deaths from cancer, and 4,259 women had hip fractures during their lifetime. Milk played a significant role in each category but not in the way you might expect.

This study looked at milk consumption and nearly one hundred other food items as well. This allowed the research staff to cross-check and to control, so they could isolate the contribution of a single item like milk to health and disease. This study controlled for medication and practices that influence bone health as well. Smoking status, cortisone use, estrogen use, and physical activity of participants were evaluated, and proper adjustments made.

In this study the amount of milk a person drank each day was measured and correlated with the likelihood of dying from coronary heart disease. Here is a graph of the results in women.

Figure 4. Heart attack deaths of Swedish women who were not Seventh-day Adventists by the number of glasses of milk drunk per day[14]
Significance = narrow 95% confidence intervals

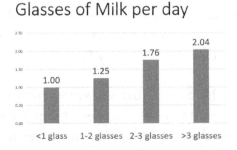

Heart Disease Deaths by Glasses of Milk per day

As the glasses of milk drunk each day increased, so did deaths from heart disease. There was a 25 percent increase with one to two glasses of milk a day. This went up to a 76 percent increase in heart disease deaths for women drinking two to three glasses of milk a day and more than doubled the risk of a heart attack for those dinking more than three glasses of milk per day.

The numbers weren't any better when it comes to cancer.

Figure 5. Cancer deaths of Swedish women who were not Seventh-day Adventists by the number of glasses of milk drunk per day[15]
Significance = narrow 95% confidence intervals

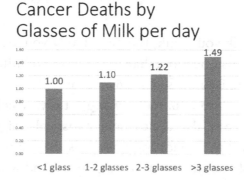

The more milk you drink, the more likely you are to die of cancer. There is a 49 percent increase in risk of cancer deaths if you drink more than three glasses of milk per day.

The calcium-rich milk is proclaimed as essential in the diet to maintain bone strength and stave off fractures of the hip in women. Unfortunately, this is a myth. Drinking milk increases the risk of hip fracture in women.

Figure 6. Hip fractures of Swedish women who were not Seventh-day Adventists by the number of glasses of milk drunk per day[16]
Significance = narrow 95% confidence intervals

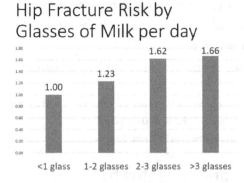

Hip Fracture Risk by
Glasses of Milk per day

	1.00	1.23	1.62	1.66
	<1 glass	1-2 glasses	2-3 glasses	>3 glasses

The more milk you drink, the more likely you are to have a hip fracture. If you consume more than three glasses of milk each day, the risk of hip fracture is increased by 66 percent.

This is just one study but a very large study, which increases its importance. There is also a clear and statistically significant dose-response relationship implicating milk. It is these kinds of data that thoughtful people can use to stop using milk. And what is the harm in discarding milk from the diet?

Thomas M. Campbell II, MD, coauthor with his father, T. Colin Campbell, of *The China Study*, has published a well-referenced list of the "12 Frightening Facts about Milk."[17]

1. In observational studies both across countries and within single populations, higher dairy intake has been linked to increased risk of prostate cancer.
2. Observational cohort studies have shown higher dairy intake is linked to higher ovarian cancer risk.
3. Cow's milk protein may play a role in triggering type 1 diabetes through a process called molecular mimicry.
4. Across countries, populations that consume more dairy have higher rates of multiple sclerosis.

5. In interventional animal experiments and human studies, dairy protein has been shown to increase IGF-1 (insulin-like growth factor-1) levels. Increased levels of IGF-1 have been implicated in several cancers.

6. In interventional animal experiments and human experiments, dairy protein has been shown to promote increased cholesterol levels (in the human studies and animal studies) and atherosclerosis (in the animal studies).

7. The primary milk protein (casein) promotes cancer initiated by a carcinogen in experimental animal studies.

8. D-galactose has been found to be pro-inflammatory and actually is given to create animal models of aging.

9. Higher milk intake is linked to acne.

10. Milk intake has been implicated in constipation and ear infections.

11. Milk is perhaps the most common self-reported food allergen in the world.

12. Much of the world's population cannot adequately digest milk due to lactose intolerance.

There are plentiful, healthful, and competitively priced alternatives to cow's milk, including soy milk, almond milk, cashew milk, rice milk, and coconut milk to mention just a few. The healthiest Seventh-day Adventists use milk sparingly if at all. Perhaps it is time for you to eliminate milk from your diet.

Every nutrient in milk can be found in whole plant foods, which is the new position endorsed by many health professionals. We are learning today that milk really isn't the "perfect food" as once thought. True, there aren't many other single foods that contain the same amount of nutrients that one gets from one cup of milk, but by eating a variety of foods, one can obtain all the necessary nutrients that milk would provide.

Milk has presented a few caveats for some, such as milk is insulinogenic in that it spikes blood sugar levels; it also has inflammatory properties, so it is a common offender of acne, sinus congestion, and digestive disorders. Because of its lactose content, many find it indigestible. Others dislike the hormones, antibiotics, and pesticides that are routinely fed to cows. Milk is one of those foods that can have a good and a bad side.

I extend thanks to the many companies that provide nutritious milk alternatives that contain many of the same nutrients as cow's milk through fortification and as grown naturally. The following graph shows a comparison of soy milk (Silk brand) with 2 percent dairy milk.

Figure 7. Comparison of Soy milk with Dairy Milk[18]

Comparison of Soy milk with Dairy Milk		
Nutrient	**Silk Original Soymilk**	**2% Dairy Milk**
Calories	110	120
Calcium	45% daily value (DV)	30% DV
Vitamin D	30% DV	25% DV
Saturated Fat	0.5 grams	3 grams
Cholesterol	0 mg	20 mg
Sugar	6 grams	12 grams
ALA Omega-3 Fatty Acids	240 mg	20 mg

Furthermore, milk is low in several nutrients: vitamin C, iron, soluble fiber, and phytochemicals.

Milk is not the only source of calcium in the diet. There are many foods that provide calcium as well. Green leafy vegetables top the list. Other calcium-rich foods include soy yogurt, fortified orange juice, tofu, okra, broccoli, green beans, almonds, and fortified soymilk. Eating foods such as these will meet the nutrient requirements for calcium.

The following graph illustrates the decline of milk consumption since 1970.

Figure 8. "Trends in U.S. Per Capita Consumption of Dairy Products, 1970-2012"[19]

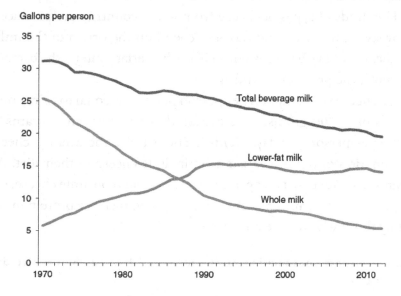

Milk availability down 37 percent since 1970

Gallons per person

Source: USDA, Economic Research Service, Food Availability (Per Capita) Data System.

The bottom line: Cow's milk is nutrient dense, with high levels of minerals, protein, vitamins, and fat. However, milk poses health risks through the health of the cow, the diet and additives in a cow's diet, the storage and delivery of milk, its lactose content, contaminants found in milk, and medical concerns related with milk consumption.

If one wishes to delete cow's milk from the diet, care should be taken to supply the same nutrients found in milk with other foods. Commercial milk like beverages are fortified to have equal amounts of most nutrients, including vitamin B12, to equal or exceed those of cow's milk.

Cheese

Cheese is a dairy product derived from milk that is produced in a wide range of flavors, textures, and forms by coagulation of the milk protein casein. It comprises proteins and fat from milk, usually the

135

milk of cows or goats. During production, the milk is usually acidified, and adding the enzyme rennet causes coagulation. The solids are separated and pressed into final form.[20]

Hundreds of types of cheese from many countries are produced. Their styles, textures, and flavors depend on the origin of the milk, whether they have been pasteurized, the butterfat content, the bacteria and mold, the processing, and aging.[21]

US cheese consumption per person per year is equal to thirty-nine pounds or 17,706 grams. This breaks down to forty-nine grams of cheese per person per day.[22] This is about twice the average cheese consumption of the Adventists who include cheese in their diet. All Seventh-day Adventist diet groups except vegans consume cheese. On the part of some, this represents an attempt to increase protein in the diet by those who don't eat flesh foods.

Figure 9. Cheese consumption of Seventh-day Adventists by the five diet category groups.[23]

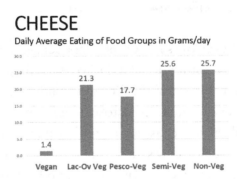

CHEESE
Daily Average Eating of Food Groups in Grams/day

Cheeses that are freshly made have nutritional qualities like the milk from which they were created. Cheeses that are aged and contain bacteria or molds become highly modified as they accumulate metabolic byproducts of the infective agents. This results in a product that is harmful to health.

Among Seventh-day Adventists who eat cheese three or more times a week, there was a 43 percent increase in breast cancer compared to those who ate cheese less than twice a month.[24]

Figure 10. Breast cancer mortality among Seventh-day Adventist Women by frequency of cheese in the diet[25]
Significance p = 0.03

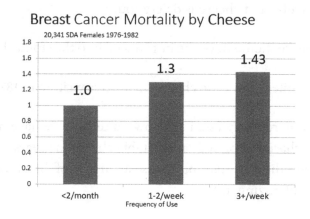

Eating cheese also had an adverse effect on the development of cancer of the ovary in Seventh-day Adventists. Postmenopausal women who ate cheese more than twice a week had twice as much ovarian cancer as women who never ate cheese or had it less than once a week.[26]

Figure 11. Risk of developing ovarian cancer in Seventh-day Adventist women by the frequency of cheese in their diet[27]
Significance p = 0.1

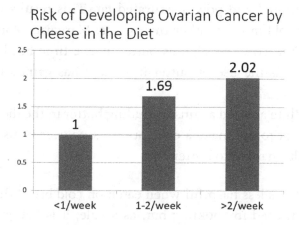

Ellen White indicated that cheese was not a healthful food item and strongly advocated for eliminating cheese from the diet.

> The effect of cheese is deleterious.[28]

> Cheese should never be introduced into the stomach.[29]

Ellen White did not use cheese. In a letter written in 1873, she said

> In regard to cheese, I am now quite sure we have not purchased or placed on our table cheese for years. We never think of making cheese an article of diet, much less of buying it.[30]

Butter

Butter is a tasty but potent source of saturated fat. Butter consumption in the United States has gradually increased over the past decade from 4.5 pounds per person per year to 5.5 pounds per person per year.[31] Margarine was designed as a replacement for butter in the middle of the last century and was initially high in saturated fat.

More recently, margarine has been engineered to contain more monounsaturated and polyunsaturated fat. This results in a softer spread now sold in tubs rather than sticks. Margarine consumption was more than twice as high as butter at one time but has slipped below butter as the use of butter in society has gained favor once again.[32]

Ellen White advised against including butter in the diet but felt it was important to not make a contentious issue over its use. She also suggested alternatives to butter.

> Butter is less harmful when eaten on cold bread than when used in cooking; but, as a rule, it is better to dispense with it altogether.[33]

We must remember that there are a great many different minds in the world, and we cannot expect everyone to see exactly as we do in regard to all questions of diet. Minds do not run in exactly the same channel. I do not eat butter, but there are members of my family who do. It is not placed on my table; but I make no disturbance because some members of my family choose to eat it occasionally.[34]

When properly prepared, olives, like nuts, supply the place of butter and flesh meats. The oil, as eaten in the olive, is far preferable to animal oil or fat.[35]

Butter is not favorably received by many Seventh-day Adventists, who consume about half the butter of the general population. It is shunned as an animal product by the vegans, and the use by lacto-ovo and pesco-vegetarians is about half that of the non-vegetarian Seventh-day Adventists.

Figure 12. Butter consumption of Seventh-day Adventists by the five diet category groups[36]

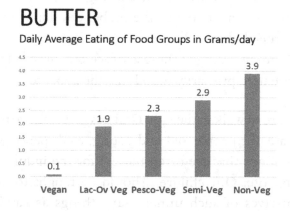

Dairy Desserts

Ice cream, ice milk, and frozen yogurt are the primary dairy desserts. Except for the vegan Seventh-day Adventists, dairy desserts are similar in consumption by the other dietary groups.

Figure 13. Dairy dessert consumption of Seventh-day Adventists by the five diet category groups[37]

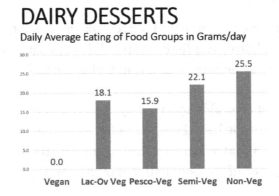

The Adventist Health Studies have not published data on the adverse health effects of dairy desserts. Ice cream is a tasty but energy-dense, high-fat, high saturated fat, and high sugar food. Ice cream consumption has contributed to the global development of obesity, diabetes, and metabolic syndrome.[38,39,40,41]

Ellen White discouraged the use of ice cream, candy, and other snacks that are used primarily to indulge the appetite.

> If we are to walk in the light God has given us, we must educate our people, old and young, to dispense with these foods that are eaten merely for the indulgence of appetite. Our children should be taught to deny themselves of such unnecessary things as candies, gum, ice cream, and other knickknacks.[42]

Small case-control studies have found an association between ice cream consumption and breast cancer,[43] lung cancer,[44] prostate cancer,[45] and deteriorating cognitive health.[46] Today, many nondairy desserts are available.

Eggs

Eggs are high in protein, but the yolk contains a great amount of cholesterol. The US government *Dietary Guidelines* states that people should eat as little dietary cholesterol as possible.[47] One extra-large, 56-gram egg contains 208mg of cholesterol, exceeding the daily recommended limit.[48]

US consumption of eggs averages forty-six grams per person per day. Seventh-day Adventists eat less eggs than the general public. Vegans eliminate eggs, and the lacto-ovo vegetarians eat half the amount of eggs as the non-vegetarian Seventh-day Adventists. The non-vegetarian Adventists eat only about one-third the amount of eggs as non-Adventists. The healthiest diet for most people does not include eggs.[49]

Figure 14. Egg consumption of Seventh-day Adventists by the five diet category groups[50]

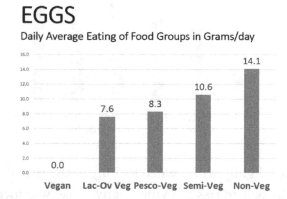

EGGS
Daily Average Eating of Food Groups in Grams/day

Because of the high cholesterol levels in eggs, scientists in the past recommended limiting the number of eggs in the diet to three a week. This disapproval of eggs has recently been questioned because the relationship between cholesterol in the diet from eggs and cholesterol in the bloodstream had not been clearly established. Persons eating eggs frequently also eat foods containing saturated fat, which raises blood cholesterol levels.

More recent data demonstrate that eggs in the diet are harmful to health.[51] One study included 29,615 participants who were not Seventh-day Adventists, of an average age of 51.6 years. The population was 44.9 percent men and 55.1 percent women. They were followed for seventeen years. During the study, there were 5,400 heart attacks and strokes, and 6,132 people died.

The risk of dying of a heart attack or stroke increased by 6 percent with each half an egg eaten per day. There was a 30 percent increase in the risk of having a heart attack or stroke for those averaging two and a half eggs per day.

Figure 15. Risk of heart attacks and strokes experienced by men and women who were not Seventh-day Adventists, by the number of eggs eaten per day[52] CI 1.03-1.10

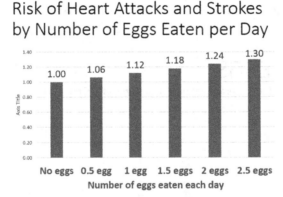

Results are slightly worse when looking at the risk of dying of all causes combined. The risk of dying of any cause was increased by 8 percent for each half egg increase in eggs eaten per day. There was a 40 percent increase in the risk of dying of any cause if eating two and a half eggs per day.

Figure 16. Risk of dying of any cause by men and women who were not Seventh-day Adventists, by the number of eggs eaten per day[53]
(CI 1.04-1.11)

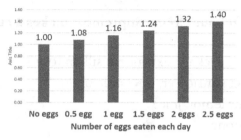

Risk of Dying of Any Cause by Number of Eggs Eaten per Day

Ellen White recommended eating eggs in certain circumstances.

> We should not consider it a violation of principle to use eggs from hens that are well cared for and suitably fed. Eggs contain properties that are remedial agencies in counteracting certain poisons.[54]

Then again, she indicated that eggs would eventually not be best for a person's health.

> But I wish to say that when the time comes that it is no longer safe to use milk, cream, butter, and eggs, God will reveal this. No extremes in health reform are to be advocated. The question of using milk and butter and eggs will work out its own problem. At present we have no burden on this line. Let your moderation be known unto all men.[55]

Discarding eggs from the diet should be reconsidered given the increase in heart attacks and strokes that has been more recently demonstrated with their use.

Recipes

For those who would like to learn a new way of eating, we invite you to experiment with some new recipes to replace milk and milk products.

Tofu Sour Crème Supreme—makes 2 cups

1 (10.5-ounce) package extra-firm silken tofu
1/4 cup olive, sunflower, or canola oil
3 tablespoons lemon juice
1 teaspoon honey
1/2 teaspoon salt

Combine all ingredients in a blender and process on high speed until smooth and creamy.

Can be used on baked potatoes, nachos, as a dip, or whenever sour cream is listed as an ingredient.

Pimento Cheez Sauce—makes 3 cups

1 cup water, divided
1/2 cup raw cashews
2 tablespoons tahini
1 and 1/2 teaspoons salt
3 tablespoons nutritional yeast flakes
2 teaspoons onion powder
1 teaspoon garlic powder
1/2 cup pimento
4 tablespoons lemon juice

Blend the cashews in 1/2 cup of the water until completely smooth. Add the rest of the water and all remaining ingredients. Mix to blend. Transfer mixture to a saucepan and cook over medium heat, stirring constantly. When mixture thickens, remove from heat. Serve warm over tortilla chips, potatoes, broccoli, cauliflower, or in any Mexican dish in place of cheese.

Tofu Cottage Cheez—makes 3 cups

1 package water-packed, extra-firm tofu
2 teaspoons onion powder
1 and 1/2 teaspoons salt
1/2 teaspoon garlic powder
2 tablespoons lemon juice
1 container (3/4 cup) Tofutti Better Than Sour Cream or homemade sour cream (see tofu sour crème supreme recipe above)

Press excess water out of tofu by squeezing the block with both hands. Place on clean, dry towel. Wrap tightly and gently squeeze to absorb the most liquid possible. Crumble tofu with hands in a bowl and add the rest of the ingredients. For variations: add chopped chives, dill, or chopped pineapple or pears.

CHAPTER 12

Preferable Protein for a Healthy Diet

Meat is getting a lot of press these days. This is because of several reasons: health concerns, environmental concerns, ethical perspectives, and economic constraints. Meat has been on the humans' menu for centuries and has become part of human traditions and cultures. It is a staple in many diets because it is a source of protein and other important nutrients. But science has uncovered many reasons why meat is not the best food for humans.

Meat is the flesh of animals and refers to the muscle or organs eaten as food. Most meat comes from domesticated animals raised on farms or large industrial complexes that house many animals. Meat can be categorized by their animal source.

1. Red meat comes from animals that contain more red blood cells in their muscle tissues. Examples include beef, pork, lamb, veal, goat, and wild game (deer, bison, and elk).
2. White meat is lighter in color than red meat and comes from fowl such as chicken, turkey, duck, goose, and wild birds (quail and pheasant). Fish is often considered a white meat.
3. Processed meat has been modified by salting, curing, smoking, drying, or other processes to preserve it or to enhance flavor or color. Examples include corned beef, frankfurters, sausage, bacon, jerky, hot dogs, and luncheon meats (bologna, salami, and pastrami).

Beef is the most popular red meat. It is typically eaten as steak, chops, ribs, roast, or ground. Red meat is more detrimental to health than white meats. Red meat can be fresh or processed. The amount of meat eaten, the type or cut of meat, the means of preparation of meat, and chemical compounds added to meat all affect a person's health. Numerous studies indicate that all forms of meat are harmful to health.

Seventh-day Adventists advocate a meat-free diet, but this recommendation is not a test of church membership. Ellen White anticipated disease and death caused by consuming meat. She also advocated the ethical treatment of animals.

> The mortality caused by eating meat is not discerned ... Animals are diseased, and by partaking of their flesh we plant the seeds of disease in our own tissues and blood.[1]

> The moral evils of a flesh diet are not less marked than are the physical ills. Flesh food is injurious to health, and whatever affects the body has a corresponding effect on the mind and the soul. Think of the cruelty to animals that meat eating involves, and its effect on those who inflict and those who behold it. How it destroys the tenderness with which we should regard these creatures of God![2]

About half of Adventists regularly eat meat. The Adventist Health Study provides compelling data showing the harmful effects of including red meat and other flesh-based food in the diet. Red meat eaten by the five subgroups of Seventh-day Adventists is seen in figure 1.[3]

Figure 1. Red meat consumption of Seventh-day Adventists by the five diet category groups[4]

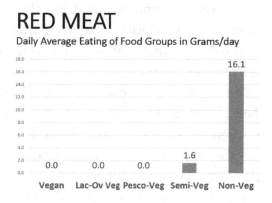

RED MEAT

Daily Average Eating of Food Groups in Grams/day

Meat and Heart Attacks

Coronary heart disease is the number one cause of death in the United States. There are multiple risk factors for heart attacks, including eating meat. This was demonstrated in the Adventist Health Study[5] and is illustrated in figure 2.

Figure 2. Risk of fatal heart attacks in Seventh-day Adventist men ages 55–64 by frequency of meat in their diet per week[6]
Significance p = 0.003

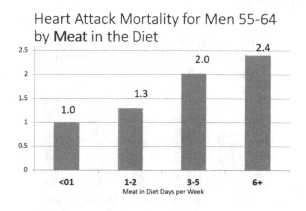

Seventh-day Adventist men eating meat six or more times a week had a 140 percent increase in the risk of fatal heart attacks compared with Seventh-day Adventists who ate meat less than once a week. There is a clear dose-response relationship demonstrated, which helps confirm the causal nature of this relationship. Eating meat increases the risk of dying from a heart attack.

Meat is extolled for its protein content. In the human digestive system, both plant and animal proteins are broken down to simple amino acids by pancreatic enzymes. Only amino acids are absorbed so as to deidentify the original protein sources that would provide an antigenic stimulus to the immune system.

Still, the source of protein has a profound effect on developing cardiovascular diseases.[7] In the AHS-2 study, the population was divided into five categories by the amount of protein in the diet and whether the protein came from meats or from nuts and seeds.

The risk of dying from heart attacks and strokes increased significantly if protein in the diet came from meats. Persons eating the highest amount of protein from meat had a 67 percent increase in the risk of dying compared to those with the lowest amount of protein in the diet from meat.

Figure 3. Risk of Seventh-day Adventist men and women dying of heart attacks or strokes by the amount of protein the diet from meat sources[8]
Significance p = <0.001

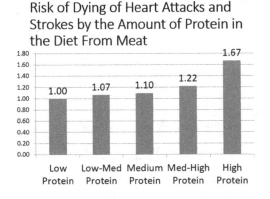

Risk of Dying of Heart Attacks and Strokes by the Amount of Protein in the Diet From Meat

The results were quite the opposite for those who got their protein from nuts and seeds. As the amount of protein in the diet of these people increased, the risk of dying of a heart attack or stroke went down. Those who ate the highest amount of protein from nuts and seeds had a 41 percent decrease in the risk of cardiovascular deaths compared to those who got the lowest amount of protein from nuts and seeds.

Figure 4. Risk of Seventh-day Adventist men and women dying of heart attacks or strokes by the amount of protein the diet from nuts and seeds[9] **Significance p = <0.001**

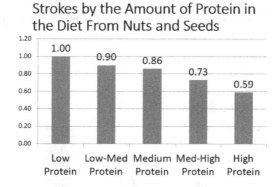

These results may not solely be because of differences in protein quality but may represent the effect of other nutrients that accompany protein in the diet. With meat there is a significant degree of saturated fat, blood, and animal hormones. Nuts and seeds are rich in unsaturated fats that are healthful, as well as fiber and other protective phytochemicals.

This evidence shows that healthy diets can include substantial amounts of protein if that protein comes from nuts and seeds, not from meat.

Meat and Cancers

Colon Cancer

In the United States, colon cancer is the number two cause of cancer death in men and the number three cause of cancer death in women.[10] In figure 5 you see the risk of developing colon cancer among Seventh-day Adventists based on the amount of red meat in their diet.[11] Seventh-day Adventists eating red meat occasionally but less than once a week had a 40 percent increase in colon cancer. Those eating red meat at least once a week had a 90 percent (almost double) risk of developing colon cancer.

Figure 5. Risk of colon cancer in Seventh-day Adventists by frequency of meat in their diet[12]
Significance p = 0.04

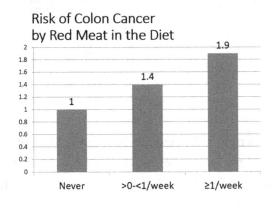

Pancreas Cancer

Another cancer associated with meat eating is cancer of the pancreas, which is the number four cause of cancer death in the United States among both men and women. In an earlier study, Seventh-day Adventists eating meat, poultry, or fish three times a week doubled their risk of dying of cancer of the pancreas.[13] This result was only of borderline significance in this study due to small numbers. A much larger study conducted later in a general population will be discussed below that confirms this early suggestion of the risk of death from pancreas cancer by eating animal products.

Figure 6. Risk of dying of cancer of the pancreas in Seventh-day Adventists by frequency of meat, poultry, and fish in their diet[14]
Significance p = 0.052

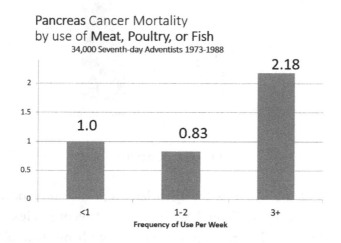

Bladder Cancer

Bladder cancer is the number four cancer to be newly diagnosed in men but is only the eighth leading cause of death due to effective treatments.[15] Bladder cancer is not in the top ten causes of cancer in women. In the Adventist Health Studies, the risk of developing bladder cancer was related to meat, poultry, and fish in the diet.[16] Those who ate meat, poultry, or fish three times a week or more experienced a more than doubling of the risk of developing bladder cancer compared to vegetarians in the study.

Figure 7. Risk of bladder cancer among Seventh-day Adventists by vegetarian and non-vegetarian diet[17]
Significance p.=0.02

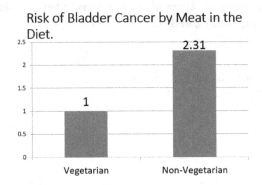

Risk of Bladder Cancer by Meat in the Diet.

Ovarian Cancer

Cancer of the ovary is the fifth leading cause of cancer deaths among women in the United States.[18] The Adventist Health Study shows a strong and significant correlation with meat, poultry, and fish in the diet of postmenopausal women.[19] Seventh-day Adventist women with flesh food in the diet once a week or more were more than twice as likely to develop ovarian cancer compared with Seventh-day Adventist women who were vegetarian.

Figure 8. Risk of ovarian cancer in Seventh-day Adventist women by meat, poultry, and fish in their diet[20]
Significance p = 0.006

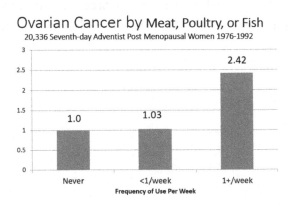

Ovarian Cancer by Meat, Poultry, or Fish
20,336 Seventh-day Adventist Post Menopausal Women 1976-1992

Meat and Diabetes

There is a wide range in the prevalence of type 2 diabetes among Seventh-day Adventists.[21] Vegan Seventh-day Adventists have only 22 percent of the diabetes of those who are non-vegetarians.

Figure 9. Relative risk of diabetes in Seventh-day Adventists by the five diet categories[22]

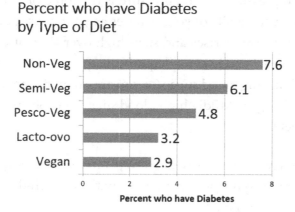

Percent who have Diabetes by Type of Diet

Percent who have Diabetes

Meat and the Metabolic Syndrome

Metabolic syndrome is the name for a group of risk factors that raises your risk for heart disease and other health problems, such as diabetes and stroke. There are five conditions described below that are metabolic risk factors. You can have any one of these risk factors by itself, but they tend to occur together. You must have at least three metabolic risk factors to be diagnosed with metabolic syndrome.[23]

1. A large waistline. This is also called abdominal obesity or "having an apple shape." Excess fat in the stomach area is a greater risk factor for heart disease than excess fat in other parts of the body, such as on the hips.

2. A high triglyceride level (or you are on medicine to treat high triglycerides). Triglycerides are a type of fat found in the blood.

3. A low HDL cholesterol level (or you are on medicine to treat low HDL cholesterol). HDL sometimes is called "good" cholesterol. This is because it helps remove cholesterol from your arteries. A low HDL cholesterol level raises your risk for heart disease.

4. High blood pressure (or you are on medicine to treat high blood pressure). Blood pressure is the force of blood pushing against the walls of your arteries as your heart pumps blood. If this pressure rises and stays high over time, it can damage your heart and lead to plaque buildup.

5. High fasting blood sugar (or you are on medicine to treat high blood sugar). Mildly high blood sugar may be an early sign of diabetes.

Seventh-day Adventists who are vegetarians have only 44 percent of the metabolic syndrome compared with Seventh-day Adventists who are not vegetarian.[24]

Meat Data from the General Population

The relationship between diet, heart disease, and cancer discovered decades ago in the Adventist Health Study was one important reason that additional research was fostered by universities and the US government in much larger populations in secular society. Were these findings of the harmful effects of flesh foods in the diet unique to Seventh-day Adventists? Would this be a finding that could be carried over into the general population?

Several large studies investigated the diet question further. One of the largest was a study funded and conducted by the US National Institutes of Health, utilizing the membership of the American Association of Retired People (NIH-AARP study). This investigation was ten times larger than the Adventist Health Study and enrolled over half a million participants followed for over ten years.

The NIH-AARP study enrolled people fifty to seventy-one years of age. Disease develops more frequently in older people, making them a preferred group to study. This study was nationwide in scope. Six states were included (California, Florida, New Jersey, North Carolina, Pennsylvania, and Louisiana) and two metropolitan areas (Detroit, Michigan, and Atlanta, Georgia).

This study enrolled 322,263 men and 223,390 women. This large pool of participants made it possible to consider many lifestyle characteristics that might confound or confuse the data. The NIH-AARP study controlled for thirty-one levels of smoking and tobacco use, five levels of physical activity, age, gender, education level, marital status, family history of cancer, obesity as measured by four levels of body mass index (BMI), five levels of alcohol use, the intake of fruits and vegetables (five levels each), and using vitamins, minerals, and herbal supplements.

One potential disadvantage in this secular study was that there are very few vegetarians in the general population. The control group against which others were measured was the segment of the population with the lowest intake of red meat. These people are still at risk. The Adventist Health study showed those who ate meat only once a week often had twice the risk of vegetarians. Because of this bias, the results of the NIH-AARP study do not look quite as bad as the data would have looked had comparisons been made with more healthy vegetarians, as found in the Adventist Health Studies.

Dozens of scientific articles have been published based on data from the NIH-AARP study looking at one dietary relationship and another with various causes of death. We will only look at the finding regarding red meat and the likelihood of dying from all causes combined—overall mortality.[25]

Figure 10. The risk of dying of any cause in men who are not Seventh-day Adventists by red meat in their diet[26]
Significance p = <0.0001

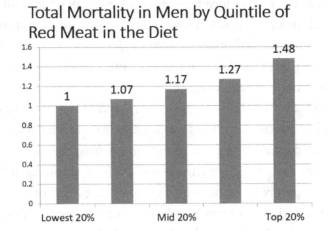

Total Mortality in Men by Quintile of Red Meat in the Diet

The men eating red meat were divided into five groups of equal size, with the group with the lowest red meat intake on the left and the group with the highest red meat intake on the right, with groups with intermediate amounts of red meat between. Each group represented about 20 percent of the study population.

The conclusion to be drawn is those with the highest intake of red meat were 48 percent more likely to die compared with those with the lowest intake of red meat. (This likely would have been a 100 percent or more increase in the chance of dying if the group with the highest intake of red meat were compared with vegetarians rather than those who simply ate less red meat.)

The numbers were even more alarming for women.

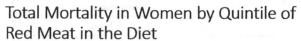

Figure 11. The risk of dying of any cause in women who are not Seventh-day Adventists by red meat in their diet[27]
Significance p = <0.0001

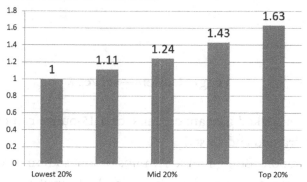

Total Mortality in Women by Quintile of Red Meat in the Diet

The women in the top 20 percent of those who ate red meat had a 63 percent increase in the risk of dying compared with the women in the bottom 20 percent of red meat intake. These numbers would have been even worse if the top 20 percent had been compared with vegetarians rather than with those with the lowest 20 percent of red meat intake.

The NIH-AARP study included so many hundreds of thousands of study subjects that the investigators discovered several associations between eating red meat and cancer. In this text we omit the graphs, but red meat was a cause of cancer of the pancreas,[28] cancer of the colon, cancer of the liver, esophageal cancer, stomach cancer, and acute myeloid leukemia.[29]

Red meat may be considered a source of complete protein but eating red meat will shorten your life by causing an increase in heart disease and several cancers.

Quiz: Rank these meats from the highest to the lowest in saturated fat per 100 grams. (Answer is at the end of this chapter.)

Rank	Food Item
	Ground beef
	Chicken
	Processed meat
	Lean beef

Recipes

Veggie Cutlets—serves 8

2 cups of soaked garbanzo beans, or a 15-ounce can of garbanzo beans drained and rinsed

2 tablespoons Bragg Liquid Aminos or low-sodium soy sauce

1/2 to 1 teaspoon liquid smoke or smoked paprika

2 tablespoons of nutritional yeast

2 tablespoons onion powder or 1/4 cup of fresh onion, chopped

1/2 teaspoon garlic powder or 1 clove of fresh garlic

1/4 cup of pecans, chopped

1/4 cup celery, chopped

3 tablespoons chicken-like seasoning or beef like-seasoning

1 and 1/2 cups water

2 and 3/4–3 and 1/2 cups of vital wheat gluten, divided

Place all above ingredients except the vital wheat gluten in a blender, and blend until smooth.

Place 2 and 3/4 cups of vital wheat gluten in a large bowl. Pour all ingredients from the blender into the vital wheat gluten in the bowl and mix well. Kneed or mix in an extra 1/2–3/4 cup of vital wheat gluten to form a stiff dough. Form into two logs and place on an oiled baking sheet and bake for 50 minutes at 350 degrees F.

Cool on rack. When cool, slice thin and simmer in broth (recipe below) for ten minutes for gluten steaks. If you want some for sandwich slices, slice thin and use as is.

Broth:

4 cups water
2 tablespoons Bragg Liquid Aminos or low-sodium soy sauce
2 tablespoons chicken-like or beef-like seasoning or Better than Bouillon Vegetable Base
1 teaspoon liquid smoke

Bulgur Meatballs—serves 8

1 cup bulgur wheat
1/2 cup soy sauce
1 box extra-firm tofu, mashed
1 tube Ritz crackers, crushed
1 onion, finely chopped
1 teaspoon sage
1 teaspoon salt
2 tablespoons nutritional yeast flakes
2 tablespoons flaxseed, ground
3 tablespoons vital wheat gluten
2 teaspoons garlic powder
1/2 cup ground walnuts

Soak the bulgur wheat overnight in water; drain in the morning. Marinate the bulgur wheat in soy sauce for 20 minutes. Drain.

Add remaining ingredients together and mix well. If mixture is too dry to form into balls, add a little soy sauce. Pinch off and roll into balls or make patties.

Bake at 350 degrees F for 45 minutes. These can be frozen.

Sweet-and-Sour Sauce—makes 2 ½ cups

1/2 cup brown sugar
1 cup ketchup
1/2 cup BBQ sauce

1–2 teaspoons soy sauce

1/2 teaspoon lemon juice

3/4 cup water

Mix and cover cooked meatballs.

Bake at 350 degrees F for 20–30 minutes.

Serve over rice, potatoes, vegetables, or in a sandwich.

Answer to the Quiz

Rank	Food Item
2	Ground beef
4	Chicken
1	Processed meat
3	Lean beef

CHAPTER 13

Other Healthful Lifestyle Factors beyond Diet

T he best nutritional strategies for a long and healthy life have been the major focus of this book. But a long life and the best of health depend on additional lifestyle elements advocated and practiced by the healthiest Seventh-day Adventists.

Nature's Resources for Health

The Seventh-day Adventists have an extensive library of historical church documents that contain the advice that results in Adventists being the healthiest people in the world. One of the most concise summaries of what it takes to be healthy is the following statement.

> Pure air, sunlight, abstemiousness, rest, exercise, proper diet, the use of water, trust in divine power— these are the true remedies. Every person should have a knowledge of nature's remedial agencies and how to apply them.[1]

Each true remedy will be briefly considered in this chapter.

Pure Air

Over the past thirty years, researchers have unearthed an array of health effects related to air pollution exposure. Among them are respiratory diseases, including asthma and changes in lung function, cardiovascular diseases, adverse pregnancy outcomes (such as preterm birth), and even death. In 2013, the World Health Organization concluded that outdoor air pollution is a carcinogen to humans.[2]

For optimum health, live where the outdoor air is clean and fresh. Avoid indoor air pollution by providing for adequate ventilation and/or filtration.

Sunlight

Most public health messages of the past century have focused on the hazards of too much sun exposure. Ultraviolet radiation penetrates deeply into the skin, where it can contribute to skin cancer. However, excessive ultraviolet exposure accounts for only 0.1 percent of the total global burden of disease according to the 2006 World Health Organization report *The Global Burden of Disease Due to Ultraviolet Radiation*.[3]

The best-known benefit of sunlight is its ability to boost the body's vitamin D supply; most cases of vitamin D deficiency are due to lack of outdoor sun exposure. At least one thousand genes governing virtually every tissue in the body are now thought to be regulated by 1,25-dihydroxyvitamin D_3, the active form of the vitamin, including several involved in calcium metabolism and neuromuscular and immune system functioning.[4]

Get some sunshine almost daily on some exposed skin, but not enough to burn.

Abstemiousness

Abstemiousness is no longer in our vocabulary, but synonyms include *sobriety, temperance, abstinence, self-control,* and *moderation.*

Things in this category that Seventh-day Adventists avoid are covered in the next chapter.

Rest

Sleep affects almost every tissue in our bodies. It affects growth and stress hormones, our immune system, appetite, breathing, blood pressure, and cardiovascular health.

Tired people are less productive at work. They are at a much higher risk for traffic accidents. Lack of sleep also influences your mood, which can affect how you interact with others. A sleep deficit over time can even put you at greater risk for developing depression.

Research shows that lack of sleep increases the risk for obesity, heart disease, and infections. Your body releases hormones during sleep that help repair cells and control the body's use of energy. These hormone changes can affect your body weight.[5]

Sleep requirements vary considerably by age.[6]

Figure 1. Recommended hours of sleep per day by age group[7]

Age Group		Recommended Hours of Sleep Per Day
Newborn	0–3 months	14–17 hours
Infant	4–12 months	12–16 hours per 24 hours (including naps)
Toddler	1–2 years	11–14 hours per 24 hours (including naps)
Preschool	3–5 years	10–13 hours per 24 hours (including naps)
School age	6–12 years	9–12 hours per 24 hours
Teen	13–17 years	8–10 hours per 24 hours
Adult	18–60 years	7 or more hours per night
	61–64 years	7–9 hours per night
	65 and older	7–8 hours per night

Seventh-day Adventists also rest one day a week in observance of the Saturday Sabbath of the Bible. On this weekly recurring day of rest, no commercial work is done except for essential services and provision of health care. The Sabbath is observed for a twenty-four-hour period from sundown on Friday until sundown on Saturday.

Exercise

The benefits of exercise are widely known but rarely pursued. Guidelines for exercise by adults have been published by the Center for Disease Control and Prevention of the US government.[8]

1. Adults should move more and sit less throughout the day. Some physical activity is better than none. Adults who sit less and do any amount of moderate-to-vigorous physical activity gain some health benefits.
2. For substantial health benefits, adults should do at least 150 minutes (two hours and thirty minutes) to three hundred minutes (five hours) a week of moderate-intensity or seventy-five minutes (one hour and fifteen minutes) to one hundred fifty minutes (two hours and thirty minutes) a week of vigorous-intensity aerobic physical activity, or an equivalent combination of moderate- and vigorous-intensity aerobic activity. Preferably, aerobic activity should be spread throughout the week.
3. Additional health benefits are gained by engaging in physical activity beyond the equivalent of three hundred minutes (five hours) of moderate-intensity physical activity per week.
4. Adults should also do muscle-strengthening activities of moderate or greater intensity and that involve all major muscle groups on two or more days per week, as these activities provide additional health benefits.

Here is an example of the advice Seventh-day Adventists received over one hundred years ago on the benefits of exercise.

> The more we exercise, the better will be the circulation of the blood. More people die for want of exercise than through overfatigue; very many more rust out than wear out. Those who accustom themselves to proper exercise in the open air will generally have a good and

vigorous circulation. We are more dependent upon the air we breathe than upon the food we eat.

Men and women, young and old, who desire health, and who would enjoy active life, should remember that they cannot have these without a good circulation. Whatever their business and inclinations, they should make up their minds to exercise in the open air as much as they can. They should feel it a religious duty to overcome the conditions of health which have kept them confined indoors, deprived of exercise in the open air.[9]

Proper Diet

Chapters 1-12 of this book have dealt with the dietary philosophy and practice of Seventh-day Adventists.

Use of Water

Water as a beverage is considered earlier in this book, but there also are benefits from the external application of water. Here is a sample of the advice Seventh-day Adventists have received on the beneficial effects of the external application of water.

In health and in sickness, pure water is one of heaven's choicest blessings. Its proper use promotes health ... The external application of water is one of the easiest and most satisfactory ways of regulating the circulation of the blood. A cold or cool bath is an excellent tonic. Warm baths open the pores and thus aid in the elimination of impurities. Both warm and neutral baths soothe the nerves and equalize the circulation.[10]

Trust in Divine Power

This last true remedy, for many Adventists, is the most important. Another reason Seventh-day Adventists are the healthiest people in the world is because God provides those who ask the power to live the life he prescribes.

A meaningful religious life can help a person cope with stress, experience less cardiovascular disease, possess an improved immune system, make fewer hospital visits, and cope with depression. These benefits have been summarized by several authors. [11,12]

Most everyone knows what they should do to maintain or recover health, but they just don't do it. Many make better choices for a while but give up too soon. Behavior change of an entire population is difficult to accomplish.

Successful Seventh-day Adventists have learned certain basic spiritual truths. Jesus said,

> I am the vine, you are the branches. He who abides in Me, and I in him, bears much fruit; for *without Me you can do nothing* (John 15:5).

The flip side of this quotation is

> *I can do all things* through Christ who strengthens me (Philippians 4:13).

The healthiest Seventh-day Adventists try to be informed about health, to have a life-enhancing strategy to pursue, and to make efforts to accomplish these goals, but they trust in God to provide the power to perform.

Here are additional selections from scripture that confirm the power of God to help humans who learn to trust in him. (Emphasis added in italics.)

> He gives *power to the weak*, and to those who have no might He *increases strength* (Isaiah 40:29).

that He would grant you, according to the riches of His glory, to be *strengthened* with might through His Spirit in the inner man (Ephesians 3:16).

Now to Him who is able to do *exceedingly abundantly* above all that we ask or think, according to the *power that works in us* (Ephesians 3:20).

Blessed is the man who *trusts* in the Lord, and whose *hope* is the Lord (Jeremiah 17:7).

Blessed be the Lord, because He has heard the voice of my supplications! The Lord is *my strength* and my shield; my heart trusted in Him, and *I am helped*; therefore my heart greatly rejoices, and with my song I will praise Him (Psalm 28:6–7).

My soul shall be satisfied as with marrow and fatness, and my mouth shall praise You with joyful lips. When I remember You on my bed, I meditate on You in the night watches. Because *You have been my help*, therefore in the shadow of Your wings I will rejoice. My soul follows close behind You; *Your right hand upholds* me (Psalm 63:5–8).

Bless the Lord, O my soul; and all that is within me, bless His holy name! Bless the Lord, O my soul, and forget not all His benefits: Who forgives all your iniquities, who *heals all your diseases*, who redeems your life from destruction, who crowns you with lovingkindness and tender mercies, who *satisfies your mouth* with good things, so that *your youth is renewed* like the eagle's (Psalm 103:1–5).

CHAPTER 14

What the Healthiest People Avoid

There is a proverbial saying that dates to 700 BC in the work of the Greek poet Hesiod, "observe due measure; moderation is best in all things",[1] This principle was reiterated by Paul in *Philippians 4:5*: "Let your moderation be known unto all men." Moderation should only apply to healthful practices, not harmful ones that should be avoided altogether.

The healthiest Seventh-day Adventists practice moderation regarding things that are good but avoid harmful habits and practices. Things to avoid completely include tobacco, alcohol, marijuana, illegal drugs, caffeinated beverages, and flesh foods.

Tobacco

Tobacco is the single greatest cause of preventable disease in the world.[2] Burning tobacco is a veritable factory of toxic chemicals that damage multiple organs throughout the body. Cancers caused by smoking include cancers of the lung, larynx, mouth, throat, esophagus, pancreas, bladder, cervix, colon, and liver, and acute myeloid leukemia.[3]

Tobacco kills more people from cardiovascular diseases than all the cancers mentioned above.[4] Tobacco is also the major cause of emphysema, chronic bronchitis, and chronic obstructive lung disease. Smoking also causes increased mortality from aneurysms and peripheral vascular disease. Added altogether, tobacco kills four hundred thousand persons prematurely each year in the United States.[5]

Seventh-day Adventists had the following advice from Ellen White first penned in 1864, exactly one hundred years before the first Surgeon General's Report on the harmful effects of tobacco use.

> Tobacco is a poison of the most deceitful and malignant kind, having an exciting, then a paralyzing influence upon the nerves of the body. It is all the more dangerous because its effects upon the system are so slow, and at first scarcely perceivable. Multitudes have fallen victims to its poisonous influence.[6]

Seventh-day Adventists smoke less than any other population group. The prevalence of smoking is less than 1 percent for all dietary groups except the non-vegetarians, where 2 percent are current smokers.[7]

Figure 1. Current cigarette smokers among Seventh-day Adventists by the five diet category groups[8]

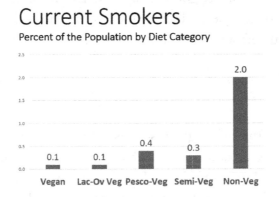

Current Smokers

Percent of the Population by Diet Category

Alcohol

Seventh-day Adventists believe the Bible advises against alcoholic beverages. The only alcoholic drinks in ancient times were wine and beer. Wine in the form of fresh grape juice is a healthful beverage and is used in religious services, including the Lord's Supper. Wine can gradually ferment and become an intoxicating beverage. The Bible discourages the use of wine that is intoxicating.

Beer must be intentionally brewed and is the "strong drink" referred to in the Bible. Beer drinking is always condemned in scripture.

> Wine is a mocker, strong drink is a brawler, and whoever is led astray by it is not wise. (Proverbs 20:1)

From their earliest history, Seventh-day Adventists were active in temperance movements. The church literature contains strong admonitions against alcoholic drinks.

> When temperance is presented as a part of the gospel, many will see their need of reform. They will see the evil of intoxicating liquors and that total abstinence is the only platform on which God's people can conscientiously stand.[9]

Alcoholic beverage consumption by Seventh-day Adventists is low.

Figure 2. Percent of Seventh-day Adventists who drink alcoholic beverages daily by the five diet groups[10]

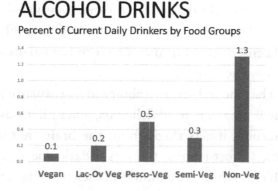

ALCOHOL DRINKS
Percent of Current Daily Drinkers by Food Groups

Vegan	Lac-Ov Veg	Pesco-Veg	Semi-Veg	Non-Veg
0.1	0.2	0.5	0.3	1.3

Because some people do not drink daily but only occasionally, a more complete picture of alcohol consumption of Seventh-day Adventists can be obtained by looking at those who *never* use alcoholic beverages.

Figure 3. The percent of Seventh-day Adventists who never drink alcoholic drinks by the five diet categories[11]

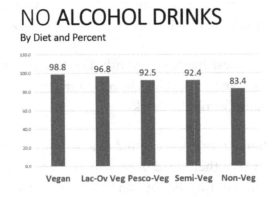

NO ALCOHOL DRINKS
By Diet and Percent

Marijuana

Marijuana for recreational use is legal in several states and for medicinal use is legal in many more states. Marijuana is most often smoked like cigarettes but is at times added to food items. Concentrates of marijuana are used for certain medical purposes.

It has not been established to what extent Seventh-day Adventists use marijuana. Adventists support the rational use of prescription medications licensed for public use. The recreational use of marijuana is discouraged by the church.

Marijuana has the well-known ability to accentuate environmental stimuli: music is amazing, food delicious, jokes hilarious, colors rich, and so on. Second, it acts throughout the brain, not just in a few targeted spots. Unfortunately, there is a dark side to all this brain stimulation. If everything is meaningful, then nothing can really stand out. Important things get lost in the blur. Without copious amounts of pot on board, everything becomes dull and uninspiring.[12] Users gradually come to lack motivation. They are less likely to graduate from high school.[13]

Figure 4. High school completion rates by frequency of marijuana use[14]

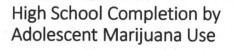

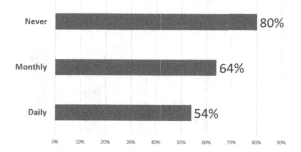

Chronic marijuana use makes the user more suitable for jobs that don't require creativity or innovation. Users become depressed and apathetic. They are also prone to psychotic breaks.

A large study looked at marijuana use and psychotic disorders in several countries, including England, France, the Netherlands, Italy, Spain, and Brazil.[15] This was a case-control study that included 901 patients ages eighteen to sixty-four who had their first psychotic disorder. These sick individuals were compared with a nonpsychotic control group carefully matched by age and geographic locality. Marijuana use in both groups was compared. The potency of the marijuana was also considered. Marijuana that contained less than 10 percent tetrahydrocannabinol (THC) was compared with marijuana containing over 10 percent THC. The frequency of marijuana use was also documented. A strong dose-response relationship between marijuana use and psychosis was documented.

Those using strong marijuana with over 10 percent THC at least once a week had a 112 percent increase in the risk of psychotic episodes compared with those who never used marijuana (risk = 2.12). Those smoking low-potency marijuana (<10 percent TCH) daily had a 208 percent increase in risk of psychotic breaks (risk = 3.08). Those smoking high-potency marijuana daily had a 481 percent increase in the risk of psychotic breaks (risk = 5.81) compared with nonusers.

Figure 5. Risk of psychotic disorder by frequency and potency of marijuana use[16]

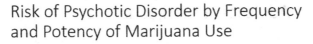
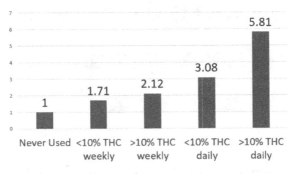

Marijuana use also leads to using illegal drugs.[17] Those who used marijuana monthly in their teen years were 3.3 times as likely to use illegal drugs as adults. Those who smoked marijuana weekly as adolescents were six times more likely to use illegal drugs as adults, and those who in their youth used marijuana daily were ten times as likely to use illegal drugs as adults.

Figure 6. Risk of adult illicit drug use by adolescent marijuana use[18]

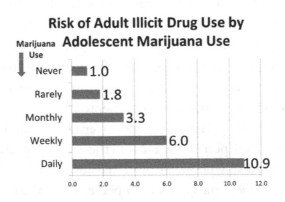

In the United States, suicide is the number two cause of death for persons ages fifteen to thirty-five.[19] There are many root causes of suicide, but chronic marijuana use is one of them. The likelihood of attempting suicide as an adult was positively correlated with the amount of marijuana smoked as an adolescent.[20]

Figure 7. Risk of adult suicide attempts by frequency of adolescent marijuana use[21]

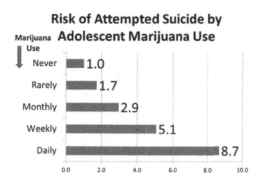

Illegal Drugs

Illegal drugs include a range of naturally occurring plants or concentrates, primarily including cocaine, opium, heroin, and some amphetamines. There are new synthetic psychoactive substances being created almost daily and sold under a wide variety of street names. Some of these chemicals are mutations of morphine, while others are synthetic amphetamines.

Carfentanil or carfentanyl is an analogue of the popular synthetic opioid analgesic fentanyl and is one of the most potent opioids known. It has a quantitative potency approximately ten thousand times that of morphine and one hundred times that of fentanyl and contributes to the death of thousands each year.[22] Synthetically derived methamphetamine is a popular drug of abuse. The church recommends complete avoidance of these natural and synthetic substances of abuse.

— CHAPTER 15 —

Practicing a Healthful Lifestyle

L iving a healthful life is easy if you were born into a family that regularly lived all the elements of a healthful lifestyle. Most are not that fortunate. First, learn how best to live, and then put it into practice. Here is an abbreviated step-by-step strategy for making lifestyle changes.

Making Healthy Changes

These suggested methods will help you make healthy changes.

1. Focus on one behavior change goal at a time.
2. Pick a behavior you do not have full control over.
3. Identify your motivation to adopt a healthy behavior. If the reason for change isn't important enough to you to make the change, pick a different behavior to tackle. Be honest.
4. Do the research. In almost every theory of healthy behavior change, knowledge is a key predictor, or at least a precursor, of successful change.
5. Give it time. Permanent changes require practice.
6. Ask for help. Professional or family help is great, but God's help is the best.

7. Change the environment in ways that will encourage your new behavior.
8. Find a buddy or join a health club or support group.
9. Work toward small and attainable goals.
10. Celebrate success. You can reward yourself as progress is being made.

The sooner you get started, the more good health you will enjoy. It is never too late to receive and enjoy the benefits of healthful living. Obviously, those living their entire lives in a healthful way will have the most to gain. But those of you who start late in life can still achieve remarkable progress. You can reverse the burden of years of disease. You can still add many healthy and enjoyable years to life.

You change slowly by making small incremental changes one at a time until you are comfortable and then go on later making more changes. This avoids the discomfort of drastic changes and a complete upset of your life. This is often the best way to make changes. Others experiencing an acute health crisis need to make drastic changes immediately. Sudden changes can be uncomfortable but can pay important health dividends quickly.

A critical issue is, can this be sustained? People often relapse into old habits and ways of living. The success of a day sometimes results in failure eventually. How can you become resistant to failure? It is possible, because a whole diverse population of Seventh-day Adventists have done it. There is no secret formula.

One clue regarding the success of Seventh-day Adventists is that all are members of a church. At one level there is singleness in belief and a sense of belonging to a caring group. The church has an articulated set of health principles presented to new members as an ideal lifestyle when they join the church.

Regular church attendance in a stable rural population is a marker for better health. Those who frequently attend church experience less heart disease, emphysema, cirrhosis of the liver, suicide, and cancer of the colon and rectum.[1] A recent national survey of church attendance confirms that church attendance results in reduced mortality.[2]

Not all Seventh-day Adventists follow the health advice of the church. Official church membership does not depend on one's adherence to the health principles of the church. But there are many millions of Seventh-day Adventists who do live healthfully. They constitute the healthiest people in the world, as research has proven.

There is more to living a healthful life than being a member of a church and knowing the health principles advocated by the church. And more to living a healthful life than the fellowship and companionship provided in a close-knit community of church people.

Seventh-day Adventists learn that God provides the power to perform. Temptations to relapse into old destructive patterns of living can be resisted by the power of God. Adventists believe that God is a personal God, who maintains a special relationship with those who become acquainted with him. God responds positively to anyone who seeks his help. The most basic and primitive call to God for help always receives a positive response.

For Seventh-day Adventists, good health is the gift of God given to those who follow the laws of healthful living by the power provided by God to those who ask for it. Success in life is all of God and none of us.

> I can do all things through Christ who strengthens me.
> (Philippians 4:13)

You need not join a church in order to live a healthful life or to receive God's help to live a healthful life. God's gift of grace is open to all who seek his help. So, don't delay. The principles of living the healthiest life possible are covered in this book. They can be put into practice immediately. You will enjoy better health almost immediately. Ask God for strength to do it. Then do it.

But if you would like to get to know the healthiest people in the world, visit a Seventh-day Adventist church some Saturday and ask to speak to the healthiest person there about healthful living. Drop in for a visit.

Healthful Living Can Work for Everyone

There are numerous studies of populations with varying degrees of good health habits that parallel the results of the Adventist Health Study. We cite one here because it offers contemporary confirmation that anyone can enjoy a healthful life if they put into practice the principles of healthful living.[3]

This study included 23,153 German participants ages thirty-five to sixty-five. Only four risk factors for disease were measured. Smokers were divided into those who never smoked and active and former smokers. Weight was divided into those with a BMI under 30 and those with a BMI 30 or higher. Physical activity was divided into those who exercised three and a half hours per week or more and those who exercised less than three and a half hours per week. Diet was divided into two groups. The positive diet group included those who ate less red meat and more fruits and vegetables. Fish and poultry were not counted, and types of bread were not considered. Those with a negative diet ate more red meat and few fruits and vegetables.

This population was followed for eight years. Persons were evaluated every two years by questionnaire to make sure which category they were in. During the study, investigators looked at developing diabetes, heart attacks, strokes, and cancer in the study population by the number of positive elements in a person's lifestyle. The results were dramatic.

The most impressive results were found with diabetes. Those with all four positive lifestyle elements had 92 percent less development of diabetes compared with those who had no positive elements in their lifestyle.

Figure 1. The risk of developing diabetes by the number of positive lifestyle elements practiced[4]
Significance: p = 0.001

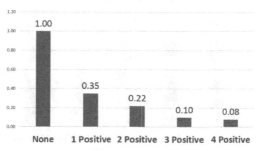

Those with four positive lifestyle practices were 81 percent less likely to have a heart attack during the study period of eight years.

Figure 2. The risk of experiencing a heart attack by the number of positive lifestyle elements practiced by the study population[5]
Significance p = <0.001

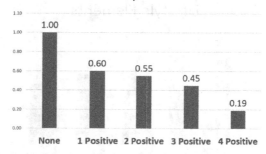

The reduction in the risk of a stroke was not as dramatic as the reduction in risk of developing diabetes or having a heart attack but was still impressive.

Figure 3. Risk of experiencing a stroke by the number of positive lifestyle elements practiced[6]
Significance: p = <.001

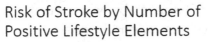
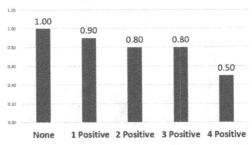

There was also a significant reduction in the risk of developing any cancer. Those who practiced all four positive factors experienced a 36 percent reduction in the risk of developing cancer.

Figure 4. The risk of developing cancer by the number of positive lifestyle elements practiced[7]
Significance: p = <0.001

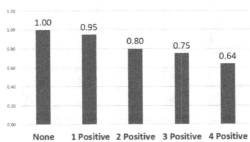

This and other similar studies are based on populations in specific geographic locations. An attempt is made to enroll as many volunteers as possible. Usually, middle-aged to older populations are chosen. Studies usually exclude all who are already sick, and some exclude any who develop disease during the first year or so of the study as these were likely to have been sick as the beginning of the study and just didn't know it.

The Adventist Health Study was different in that they attempted to enroll all Seventh-day Adventists in North America. Participants came from across the nation—from towns and cities large and small. All were members of the Seventh-day Adventist church, which advocates a healthful lifestyle. Some members do this well and have been doing it all their lives.

We have shown you the best possible way to live based on sound scientific data. With God's help you can live right and improve or regain health. Now, go and do it.

ENDNOTES

Introduction

1   Ellen G. White, "Selection of Food" *Ministry of Healing* (1905), 296.

Chapter 1. Who Are the Healthiest People?

1   Michael J. Orlich et al., "Patterns of Food Consumption among Vegetarians and Non-Vegetarians," *British Journal of Nutrition* 112, no. 10 (November 2014): 1644–53.

2   Figure 1 was created by the author based on data from the study cited in endnote 1.

3   Jean L. Schlienger, "Type 2 Diabetes Complications," *Presse Medicine* 42, no. 5 (May 2013): 839–48. [Article in French.]

4   Gary E. Fraser, "Vegetarian Diets: What Do We Know of Their Effects on Common Chronic Diseases?" *American Journal of Clinical Nutrition* 89 (2009): 1607S-1612S.

5   Figure 2 was created by the author based on data from the study cited in endnote 4

6   High Blood Pressure, U.S. Department of Health & Human Services, National Heart Lung and Blood Institute, accessed October 20, 2019, https://www.nhlbi.nih.gov/health-topics/high-blood-pressure.

7   Gary E. Fraser, "Vegetarian Diets: What Do We Know of Their Effects on Common Chronic Diseases?" *American Journal of Clinical Nutrition* 89 (2009): 1607S-1612S.

8   Figure 3 was created by the author based on data from the study cited in endnote 7.

9   2018 Obesity Maps, Centers for Disease Control and Prevention, https://www.cdc.gov/obesity, accessed October 20, 2019

10 Marie Ng, et al., "Global, Regional, and National Prevalence of Overweight and Obesity in Children and Adults during 1980–2013: A Systematic Analysis for the Global Burden of Disease Study 2013," *Lancet* 384, no. 9954 (August 30, 2014): 766–81.

11 Krista M. C. Cline and Kenneth. F. Ferraro, "Does Religion Increase the Prevalence and Incidence of Obesity in Adulthood?" *Journal for the Scientific Study of Religion* 45, no. 2 (2006): 269–81.

12 Gary E. Fraser, "Vegetarian Diets: What Do We Know of Their Effects on Common Chronic Diseases?" *American Journal of Clinical Nutrition* 89 (2009): 1607S-1612S.

13 Figure 4 was created by the author based on data from the study cited in endnote 12

Chapter 2. Why the Healthiest People Live Longer

1 Infoplease, Life Expectancy for Countries accessed October 20, 2019 https://www.infoplease.com/world/health-and-social-statistics/life-expectancy-countries-0

2 Life Expectancy, Centers for Disease Control and Prevention accessed October 20, 2019, https://www.cdc.gov/nchs/fastats/life-expectancy.htm

3 Frank. R. Lemon et al., "A Biologic Cost of Smoking, Decreased Life Expectancy," *Archives of Environmental Health* 18 (June 1969): 950–55.

4 Figure 1 was created by the author based on data from the study cited in endnote 3.

5 Figure 2 was created by the author based on data from the study cited in endnote 3.

6 Vinjar. Fonnebo, "Mortality in Norwegian Seventh-day Adventists 1962–1986," *Journal of Clinical Epidemiology* 1992, 45, no. 2, 157–167.

7 Figure 3 was created by the author based on data from the study cited in endnote 6.

8 J. Berkel and F. de Waard, "Mortality Pattern and Life Expectancy of Seventh-day Adventists in the Netherlands," *The International Journal of Epidemiology* 12 (1983): 455–59.

9 Figure 4 was created by the author based on data from the study cited in endnote 8.

10 Takeshi Hirayama, "Mortality in Japanese with Life-styles Similar to Seventh-day Adventists: Strategy for Risk Reduction by Life-style Modification, *National Cancer Institute Monograph* 69 (December 1985): 143–53.

11 Figure 5 was created by the author based on data from the study cited in endnote 10.

12   Wieslaw. Jedrychowski et al., "Survival Rates among Seventh-day Adventists Compared with the General Population in Poland," *Scandinavian Journal of Social Medicine* 13 (1985): 49–52.

13   Ivar. Heuch et al., "A Cohort Study Found that Earlier and Longer Seventh-day Adventist Church Membership Was Associated with Reduced Male Mortality," *Journal of Clinical Epidemiology* 58 (2005): 83–91.

14   Ellen G. White, "The Reward of Temperance" *Youths Instructor,* July 9, 1903

15   The 10 Best Foods For Longevity, verywell Health, accessed October 20, 2019, https://www.verywellhealth.com/best-foods-for-longevity-4005852

16   Emanuele Di Angelantonio et.al, "Body-mass Index and All-Cause Mortality: Individual-Participant-Data Meta-Analysis of 239 Prospective Studies in Four Continents," *Lancet* 388, no. 10046 (August 20, 2016): 776–86.

17   Cari M. Kitahara et al., "Association between Class III Obesity and Mortality," *PLOS Medicine* July 8, 2014.

18   Michael Miller and William. F. Fry, "The Effect of Mirthful Laughter on the Human Cardiovascular System," *Medical Hypotheses* 73, no. 5 (November 2009): 636.

19   Toshihiko Maruta et al., "Optimists vs. Pessimists: Survival Rate among Medical Patients over a 30-Year Period," *Mayo Clinic Proceedings* 75, no. 2 (February 2000): 140–43.

20   Becca R. Levy, et, al, "Longevity Increased by Positive Self-perceptions of Aging" *Journal of Personality and Social Psychology,* 2002, Aug:83 (2) 261-270.

21   Karina. W. Davidson, et.al, "Don't worry, be happy: positive affect and reduced 10-year incident coronary heart disease: The Canadian Nova Scotia Health Survey" *European Heart Journal* (2010) 31, 1065–1070

22   Ellen G. White, Chap. 18 - Mind Cure, *Ministry of Healing* (1905) 241

23   Rebecca L. Siegel, *et. al.* Cancer Statistics, 2017, *CA A Cancer Journal for Clinicians,* Vol 67:7-30.

24   Smoking and Tobacco Use, Tobacco Related Mortality, Center for Disease Control and Prevention, accessed October 20, 2019 https://www.cdc.gov/tobacco/data_statistics/fact_sheets/health_effects/tobacco_related_mortality/

25   Deborah Kotz, "11 Health Habits that will Help You Live to 100" U.S. News Health/Family Health, accessed October 22, 2019 https://health.usnews.com/health-news/family-health/living-well/articles/2009/02/20/10-health-habits-that-will-help-you-live-to-100

26   Socrates, (Greek philosopher in Athens (469 BC - 399 BC)) quoted from "Plutarch, How a Young Man Ought to Hear Poems" *Plutarch's Morals.* Translated from the Greek by Several Hands. Corrected and Revised by William W. Goodwin, with an Introduction by Ralph Waldo Emerson. 5 Volumes. (Boston: Little, Brown, and Co., 1878).

Chapter 3. Fabulous Citrus Fruit

1   Michael J. Orlich et al., "Patterns of Food Consumption among Vegetarians and Non-Vegetarians," British Journal of Nutrition 112, no. 10 (November 2014): 1644–53.

2   Figure 1 was created by the author based on data from the study cited in endnote 1.

3   Ellen G. White "Educate the People" Vol. 7 Testimonies for the Church 134, August 20, 1902.

4   Figure 2 was created by the author based on data from the study cited in endnote 1.

5   Paul K. Mills, et. al, "Cohort Study of Diet, Lifestyle, and Prostate Cancer in Adventist Men," Cancer, 1989, 64:598-604.

6   Figure 3 was created by the author based on data from the study cited in endnote 5.

7   Rebecca L. Segal, et.al, "Cancer Statistics 2017" Ca A Journal for Physicians, Vol 67, No 1, January/February 2017, 7-30.

8   Mayo Clinic, Patient Care & Health Information/Diseases & Conditions/ Bladder cancer accessed on October 22, 2019 http://www.mayoclinic.org/ diseases-conditions/bladder-cancer/basics/risk-factors/con-20027606

9   Song-Yi Park, et. al. "Fruit and Vegetable Intakes are Associates with Lower Risk of Bladder Cancer among Women In Multiethnic Cohort Study", The Journal of Nutrition 2013, 1283-1292.

10 Figure 4 was created by the author based on data from the study cited in endnote 9.

11 Figure 5 was created by the author based on data from the study cited in endnote 9.

12 Ping-Ping Bao, et. al. "Fruit, Vegetable, and Animal Food Intake and Beast Cancer Risk by Hormone Receptor Status," Nutrition and Cancer August 2012, 64(6): 806-819.

13 Figure 6 was created by the author based on data from the study cited in endnote 12

14 Anqiang Wang, et. al. "Citrus Fruit Intake Substantially Reduces the Risk of Esophageal Cancer. A Meta-Analysis of Epidemiologic Studies." Medicine October 2015 94:39

15 Mayo Clinic, Patient Care and Health Information, Diseases and Conditions, Esophageal Cancer, accessed on October 22, 2019, https://www.mayoclinic. org/diseases-conditions/esophageal-cancer/symptoms-causes/syc-20356084

16 Anqiang Wang, et. al. "Citrus Fruit Intake Substantially Reduces the Risk of Esophageal Cancer. A Meta-Analysis of Epidemiologic Studies." Medicine October 2015 94:39

17   Figure 7 was created by the author based on data from the study cited in endnote 16

18   Stephanie A. Smith-Warner et. al. "Fruits, Vegetables and Lung Cancer: a Pooled Analysis of Cohort Studies," *International Journal of Cancer* 2003, 107:1001-1011.

19   Figure 8 was created by the author based on data from the study cited in endnote 18.

20   Kenneth D. Kochanek, et.al, "Deaths: Final Data for 2014," *National Vital Statistic Reports* Vol 65, No. 4, June 30, 2016, 1-122.

21   U.S. Department of Health & Human Services, National Heart Lung and Blood Institute, "The Heart Truth," accessed on October 22, 2019, https://www.nhlbi.nih.gov/health/educational/hearttruth/lower-risk/risk-factors.htm

22   Shilpa N. Bhuparthiraju et. al. "Quantity and variety in fruit and vegetable intake and risk of coronary heart disease," *American Journal of Clinical Nutrition* 2013; 98:1514-1523.

23   Figure 9 was created by the author based on data from the study cited in endnote 22.

24   Figure 10 was created by the author based on data from the study cited in endnote 22.

25   Christine Economos, and William D. Clay "Nutritional and health benefits of citrus fruits," *Agriculture and Consumer Protection* FAO, accessed October 22, 2019. http://www.fao.org/3/x2650t/x2650t03.htm.

26   Statista, Consumer Goods & FMCG, Food & Nutrition, accessed October 22, 2019, https://www.statista.com/statistics/257189/per-capita-consumption-of-fresh-citrus-fruit-in-the-us

Chapter 4. Apples, Pears, Berries, and Dried Fruit

1   Michael. J. Orlich et al., "Patterns of Food Consumption among Vegetarians and Non-Vegetarians," *British Journal of Nutrition* 112, no. 10 (November 2014): 1644–53.

2   Figure 1 was created by the author based on data from the study cited in endnote 1.

3   Ellen G. White *Letter 5, 1870,* reprinted in *Counsels on Diet and Foods* 312 (1938)

4   Ellen G. White, *Letter 363, 1907,* reprinted in *Counsels on Diet and Foods 324* (1938)

5   Figure 2 was created by the author based on data from the study cited in endnote 1.

6   Aleksandra S. Kristo et al., "Protective Role of Dietary Berries in Cancer," *Antioxidants* October 19, 2016: 1–31.

7   Sona Skrovankova et al., "Bioactive Compounds and Antioxidant Activity in Different Types of Berries," *International Journal of Molecular Sciences* 16 (2015): 24637–706.

8   Roycelynn A. Mentor-Marcel et al., "Plasma Cytokines as Potential Response Indicators to Dietary Freeze-Dried Black Raspberries in Colorectal Cancer Patients," *Nutrition and Cancer* 64, no. 6 (August 2012): 820–25.

9   Tong Chen et al., "Randomized Phase II Trial of Lyophilized Strawberries in Patients with Dysplastic Precancerous Lesions of the Esophagus," *Cancer Prevention Research* 5, no. 1 (January 2012): 41–50.

10   Jie Zheng et al., "Effects and Mechanisms of Fruit and Vegetable Juices on Cardiovascular Diseases," *International Journal of Molecular Sciences*, 18, no. 555 (2017): 15 pages.

11   Sarah A. Johnson et al., "Daily Blueberry Consumption Improves Blood Pressure and Arterial Stiffness in Postmenopausal Women with Pre- and Stage 1-Hypertension: A Randomized, Double-Blind, Placebo-Controlled Clinical Trial," *Journal of Academy of Nutrition and Dietetics* 115, no. 3 (March 2015): 369–77.

12   Arpita Basu et al., "Freeze-Dried Strawberries Lower Serum Cholesterol and Lipid Peroxidation in Adults with Abdominal Adiposity and Elevated Serum Lipids," *Journal of Nutrition* 144, no. 6 (June 2014): 830–37.

13   Torunn E. Tjelle et al., "Polyphenol-Rich Juices Reduce Blood Pressure Measures in a Randomized Controlled Trial in High Normal and Hypertensive Volunteers," *British Journal of Nutrition*, 114, no. 7 (October 14, 2015): 1054–63.

14   Arpita Basu et al., "Blueberries Decrease Cardiovascular Risk Factors in Obese Men and Women with Metabolic Syndrome," *Journal of Nutrition* 140, no. 9 (September 2010): 1582–87.

15   Arpita Basu and T. J. Lyons, "Strawberries, Blueberries, and Cranberries in the Metabolic Syndrome: Clinical Perspectives," *Journal of Agricultural Food Chemistry* 60, no. 23 (June 2012): 5687–92,

16   Iris Erlund et al., "Favorable Effects of Berry Consumption on Platelet Function, Blood Pressure, and HDL Cholesterol," *American Journal of Clinical Nutrition* 87, no. 2 (February 2008): 323–31.

17   Jace Schell et al., "Cranberries Improve Postprandial Glucose Excursions in Type 2 Diabetes," *Food Function* 8, no. 9 (September 20, 2017): 3083–90.

18   Monica L. Castro-Acosta et al., "Drinks Containing Anthocyanin-Rich Blackcurrant Extract Decrease Postprandial Blood Glucose, Insulin and Incretin Concentrations," *Journal of Nutritional Biochemistry* 38 (December 2016): 154–61.

19   Riitta Torronen et al., "Berries Reduce Postprandial Insulin Responses to Wheat and Rye Breads in Healthy Women," *Journal of Nutrition* 143, no. 4 (April 2013): 430–36.

20 Riitta. Torronen et al., "Postprandial Glucose, Insulin, and Free Fatty Acid Responses to Sucrose Consumed with Blackcurrants and Lingonberries in Healthy Women," *American Journal of Clinical Nutrition* 96, no. 3 (September 2012): 527–33.

21 Anne Nilsson et al., "Effects of a Mixed Berry Beverage on Cognitive Functions and Cardiometabolic Risk Markers; A Randomized Cross-over Study in Healthy Older Adults," *PLOS One* November 15, 2017: 1–22.

22 Sundus Khalid et al., "Effects of Acute Blueberry Flavonoids on Mood in Children and Young Adults," *Nutrients* 9, no. 2 February 20, 2017.

23 Ellen G. White, *Letter 166* (1903)

24 Ellen G. White, Chapter-12 "Help for the Homeless and the Unemployed", *Ministry of Healing 299* (1905)

25 Hosea 3:1, 1 Samuel 25:18, 30:12, Isaiah 16:7.

26 Judy A Harrison, Elizabeth L. Andress, Preserving Food: Drying Fruits and Vegetables, *University of Georgia Cooperative Extension Service*, College of Family and Consumer Sciences 2000, 1-12.

27 Figure 3 was created by the author based on data from the study cited in endnote 1.

28 Paul K. Mills, et.al., Dietary Habits and Past Medical History as Related to Fatal Pancreas Cancer Risk Among Adventists, *Cancer*, 1988, 61: 2587-2585

29 Figure 4 was created by the author based on data from the study cited in endnote 28

30 Paul K. Mills, et.al, Cohort Study of Diet, Lifestyle, and Prostate Cancer in Adventist Men, *Cancer* 1989 64:598-604

31 Figure 5 was created by the author based on data from the study cited in endnote 30

32 Ellen G. White, "Chapter-23 Diet and Health" *Ministry of Healing 299* (1905)

Chapter 5. Vegetables: Foundation Foods of a Healthy Diet

1 Ellen G. White, Letter April 29, 1896 and reprinted in Vol. 21 Manuscript Releases 6 (1990)

2 Michael J. Orlich et al., "Patterns of Food Consumption among Vegetarians and Non-Vegetarians," *British Journal of Nutrition* 112, no. 10 (November 2014): 1644–53.

3 Figure 1 was created by the author based on data from the study cited in endnote 2.

4 Victoria Miller et al., "Fruit, Vegetable, and Legume Intake, and Cardiovascular Disease and Deaths in 18 Countries (PURE): A Prospective Cohort Study", *Lancet* 390 (November 4, 2017): 2037–49.

5   Figure 2 was created by the author based on data from the study cited in endnote 4.

6   National Cancer Institute, About Cancer, "Cruciferous Vegetables and Cancer Prevention," accessed on October 23, 2019 https://www.cancer.gov/about-cancer/causes-prevention/risk/diet/cruciferous-vegetables-fact-sheet

7   National Cancer Institute, About Cancer, "Cruciferous Vegetables and Cancer Prevention," accessed on October 23, 2019 https://www.cancer.gov/about-cancer/causes-prevention/risk/diet/cruciferous-vegetables-fact-sheet

8   John D. Hayes, et.al, "The Cancer Chemopreventive Actions of Phytochemicals Derived from Glucosinolates, *European Journal of Nutrition* 47 Suppl 2 (2008): 73–88.

9   National Cancer Institute, About Cancer, "Cruciferous Vegetables and Cancer Prevention," accessed on October 23, 2019 https://www.cancer.gov/about-cancer/causes-prevention/risk/diet/cruciferous-vegetables-fact-sheet

10   Jane V. Higdon et al, "Cruciferous Vegetables and Human Cancer Risk: Epidemiologic Evidence and Mechanistic Basis," *Pharmacological Research 55*, no. 3 (March 2007): 224–36.

11   Figure 3 was created by the author based on data from the study cited in endnote 2.

12   Ellen G. White, *Letter 31, 1901* republished in *Counsels on Diet and Foods 323* (1938).

13   Ellen G. White, *Letter 6b, 1880* published in *Vol. 20 Manuscript Releases 297*

14   Michael J. Orlich et al., "Patterns of Food Consumption among Vegetarians and Non-Vegetarians," *British Journal of Nutrition* 112, no. 10 (November 2014): 1644–53.

15   Figure 4 was created by the author based on data from the study cited in endnote 14.

16   Michael J. Orlich et al., "Patterns of Food Consumption among Vegetarians and Non-Vegetarians," *British Journal of Nutrition* 112, no. 10 (November 2014): 1644–53.

17   Figure 5 was created by the author based on data from the study cited in endnote 16.

18   *USDA National Nutrient Database for Standard Reference Release 28*, May 2016, Basic Report 11356 and 11359.

19   Ellen G. White, *Letter 322, 1905* reprinted in *Counsels on Diet and Foods 323* (1938)

20   *USDA National Nutrient Database for Standard Reference Release Legacy* April 2018, Full Report 11510 Sweet Potato, cooked, boiled, without skin.

21   *USDA National Nutrient Database for Standard Reference Release Legacy* April 2018 Full Report 11367 Potatoes, boiled, cooked without skin, without salt.

22   Figure 6 was created by the author based on data from the study cited in endnote 16.

23 The World's Healthiest Foods, "What's New and beneficial about Tomatoes?" accessed October 23, 2019, www.whfoods.com/genpage. php?tname=foodspice&dbid=44.

24 Figure 6 was created by the author based on data from the study cited in endnote 16.

25 Ellen G. White, *Letter 201* (1907) published in *Vol. 7 Manuscript Releases 119* (1975)

26 Ellen G. White, *Letter 127, 1904,* reprinted in *Counsels on Diet and Foods 491* (1938)

27 Fatemeh Kiani et al., "Dietary Risk Factors for Ovarian Cancer: The Adventist Health Study (United States)," *Cancer Causes and Control* 17 (2006): 137–46.

28 Figure 8 was created by the author based on data from the study cited in endnote 27.

29 The American Cancer Society, About Ovarian Cancer, "Key Statistics for Ovarian Cancer," accessed October 23, 2019 https://www.cancer.org/cancer/ ovarian-cancer/about/key-statistics.html.

Chapter 6. Salads: The Healthy Way to Go

1 Michael J. Orlich et al., "Patterns of Food Consumption among Vegetarians and Non-Vegetarians," British Journal of Nutrition 112, no. 10 (November 2014): 1644–53.

2 Figure 1 was created by the author based on data from the study cited in endnote 1.

3 Harold A. Kahn, et.al., Association Between Reported Diet and All-Cause Mortality: Twenty-one Year Follow-up on 27,530 Adult Seventh-day Adventists, **American Journal of Epidemiology**, 1984, Vol 119, No 5, p 775-787

4 Figure 2 was created by the author based on data from the study cited in endnote 3.

5 Michael J. Orlich et al., "Patterns of Food Consumption among Vegetarians and Non-Vegetarians," *British Journal of Nutrition* 112, no. 10 (November 2014): 1644–53.

6 Figure 3 was created by the author based on data from the study cited in endnote 5.

7 Mark L. Dreher and Adrienne J. Davenport, "Hass Avocado Composition and Potential Health Effects," *Critical Reviews in Food Science and Nutrition 53*, no. 7 (May 2013): 738–50.

8 Michael J. Orlich et al., "Patterns of Food Consumption among Vegetarians and Non-Vegetarians," *British Journal of Nutrition* 112, no. 10 (November 2014): 1644–53.

9 Figure 4 was created by the author based on data from the study cited in endnote 8.

Chapter 7. Healthy People Go Nuts

1   Michael J. Orlich et al., "Patterns of Food Consumption among Vegetarians and Non-Vegetarians," British Journal of Nutrition 112, no. 10 (November 2014): 1644–53

2   Figure 1 was created by the author based on data found in endnote 1.

3   Figure 2 was created by the author based on data found in endnote 1

4   National Peanut Board, "Who Invented Peanut Butter?" accessed on October 23, 2019, http://www.nationalpeanutboard.org/peanut-info/who-invented-peanut-butter.htm.

5   M. J. Orlich et al., "Patterns of Food Consumption among Vegetarians and Non-Vegetarians," British Journal of Nutrition 112, no. 10 (November 2014): 1644–53

6   Figure 3 was created by the author based on data found in endnote 5.

7   Gary. E. Fraser et al., "A Possible Protective Effect of Nut Consumption on Risk of Coronary Heart Disease: The Adventist Health Study," Archives of Internal Medicine 1992, 133: 1416–24.

8   Gary. E. Fraser, "Nut Consumption, Lipids, and Risk of a Coronary Event," Clinical Cardiology 22 Supplement III (1999): 11–15.

9   Figure 4 was created by the author based on data found in endnote 7.

10   Figure 5 was created by the author based on data found in endnote 7.

11   Figure 6 was created by the author based on data found in endnote 7.

12   Figure 7 was created by the author based on data found in endnote 7.

13   Figure 8 was created by the author based on data found in endnote 7.

14   Figure 9 was created by the author based on data found in endnote 7.

15   Figure 10 was created by the author based on data found in endnote 7.

16   Figure 11 was created by the author based on data found in endnote 7.

17   Ellen G. White, "Chapter 23 Diet and Health," Ministry of Healing 298 (1905)

18   F. B. Hu and M. J. Stampfer, "Nut Consumption and Risk of Coronary Heart Disease: A Review of Epidemiologic Evidence," Current Atherosclerosis Reports 1 (1999): 204–09.

19   Gary E. Fraser and D. J. Shavlik, Ten years of life: Is it a matter of Choice? **Archives of Internal Medicine.** 2001, **161** (13): 1645–1652.

20   EATBYDATE "how Long Do Nuts Last?" accessed October 23, 2019, http://www.eatbydate.com/proteins/nuts/how-long-do-nuts-last-shelf-life-expiration-date/

21   Figure 12 was created by the author based on data found at the U.S. Department of Agriculture, Food Data Central, accessed October 23, 2019, https://fdc.nal.usda.gov/fdc-app.html#/?query=nuts

Chapter 8. Legumes: A Must for Healthy People

1   Michael J. Orlich et al., "Patterns of Food Consumption among Vegetarians and Non-Vegetarians," British Journal of Nutrition 112, no. 10 (November 2014): 1644–53

2   Figure 1 was created by the author based on data found in endnote 1.

3   Rebecca L. Siegel et al., "Cancer Statistics, 2017," CA A Cancer Journal for Clinicians 67 (2017): 7–30.

4   Pramil N. Singh and Gary E. Fraser, "Dietary Risk Factors for Colon Cancer in a Low-risk Population," American Journal of Epidemiology 148, no. 8 (1998): 761–74.

5   Figure 2 was created by the author based on data found in endnote 4.

6   Rebecca L. Siegel et al., "Cancer Statistics, 2017," CA A Cancer Journal for Clinicians 67 (2017): 7–30.

7   Paul K. Mills et al., "Dietary Habits and Past Medical History as Related to Fatal Pancreas Cancer Risk among Adventists," Cancer 61, no. 12 (1988): 2578–85.

8   Figure 3 was created by the author based on data found in endnote 7.

9   Paul K. Mills et al., "Cohort Study of Diet, Lifestyle, and Prostate Cancer in Adventist Men," Cancer 64, no. 3 (1989): 598–604.

10   Figure 4 was created by the author based on data found in endnote 9.

11   CDC.gov, Home and Recreational Safety, "Hip Fractures Among Older Adults" accessed November 4, 2019 https://www.cdc.gov/homeandrecreationalsafety/ falls/adulthipfx.html

12   Vichuda Lousuebsakul-Matthews et al., "Legumes and Meat Analogues Consumption Are Associated with Hip Fracture Risk Independently of Meat Intake among Caucasian Men and Women: The Adventist Health Study-2," Public Health Nutrition 10, no. 1017 (September 2013): 11pages.

13   Figure 5 was created by the author based on data found in endnote 12.

14   Donna M. Winham et al., "Pinto Bean Consumption Reduces Biomarkers for Heart Disease Risk," Journal of the American College of Nutrition 26, no. 3 (June 2007): 243–49.

15   Juscelino Tovar et al., "Combining Functional Features of Whole-grain and Legumes for Dietary Reduction of Cardiometabolic Risk: A randomized Cross-over Intervention in Mature Women," British Journal of Nutrition 111, no. 4 (February 2014): 706–14.

16   Afsaneh Bakhtiary et al., "Effects of Soy on Metabolic Biomarkers of Cardiovascular Disuse in Elderly Women with Metabolic Syndrome," Archives of Iranian Medicine 15, no. 8 (August 2012): 462–68.

17   J. W. Anderson et al., "Serum Lipid Response of Hypercholestrolemic Men to Single and Divided Doses of Canned Beans," American Journal of Clinical Nutrition 51, no. 6 (June 1990): 1013–19.

18   Saman Abeysekara et al., "A Pulse-Based Diet Is Effective for Reducing Total and LDL-Cholesterol in Older Adults," *British Journal of Nutrition* 108 Supplement 1 (August 2012): S1-3-110.

19   Figure 6 was created by the author based on data found in endnotes 14-18.

20   Somayeh Hosseinpour-Niazi et al., "Non-Soya Legume-based Therapeutic Lifestyle Change Diet Reduces Inflammatory Status in Diabetic Patients: A Randomized Cross-over Clinical Trial," *British Medical Journal* 114, no. 2 (July 2015): 213–229.

21   Figure 7 was created by the author based on data found in endnote 20.

22   Anne Nilsson et al., "Effects of Brown Beans Evening Meal on Metabolic Risk Markers and Appetite Regulating Hormones at Subsequent Standardized Breakfast: A Randomized Cross-Over Study," *PLOS One* 8, no. 4 (April 2013): p. 1–10.

23   Figure 8 was created by the author based on data found in endnote 22.

24   Ellen G. White, "Chap. 74 - Our Camp Meetings," *Vol. 2 Testimonies for the Church 602* (1870)

25   Ellen G. White, "Establish No One Rule," *Manuscript 15, 1889* reprinted in Vol. 3 Selected Messages 294.

26   United States Department of Agriculture, Dietary Guidelines for Americans 2005, "Chapter 5 – Food Groups To Encourage" accessed November 4, 2019, https://health.gov/dietaryguidelines/dga2005/document/html/chapter5.htm

Chapter 9. Fiber: Nature's Medicine

1   Jonathan W. DeVries et.al, "The Definition of Dietary Fiber," Cereal Foods World 46, no. 3 (March 2001): 112–25.

2   Andrew B. Shreiner, et.al, The gut microbiome in health and in disease. *Current opinion in gastroenterology, 31(1),* (2015) 69–75.

3   Magnus Nilsson et al., "Lifestyle Related Risk Factors in the Aetiology of Gastro-Oesophageal Reflux," *Gut* 53 (2004): 1730–35.

4   Helen G. Coleman et al., "Dietary Fiber and the Risk of Precancerous Lesions and Cancer of the Esophagus: A Systematic Review and Meta-analysis," *Nutrition Reviews* 71, no. 7 (April 24, 2013): 474–82.

5   Roberto B. Canani et al., "Potential Beneficial Effects of Butyrate in Intestinal and Extraintestinal Diseases," *World Journal of Gastroenterology*, March 28, 2011.

6   Mervyn G. Hardinge et al., "Nutritional Studies of Vegetarians, III. Dietary Levels of Fiber," *The American Journal of Clinical Nutrition* 6, no. 5 (September/October 1958): 523–25.

7   Figure 1 was created by the author based on data found in endnote 6.

8   J. K. Ross et al., "Dietary and Hormonal Evaluation of Men and Different Risks for Prostate Cancer: Fiber Intake, Excretion, and Composition, with in Vitro Evidence for an Association between Steroid Hormones and Specific Fiber Components, *American Journal of Clinical Nutrition* 51 (1990); 365–70.

9   Figure 2 was created by the author based on data found in endnote 8.

10   Yesenia Tantamango et al., "Association between Dietary Fiber and Incident Cases of Colon Polyps: The Adventist Health Study," *Gastrointestinal Cancer Research* 4, no. 5–6 (September–December 2011): 161–67.

11   Figure 3 was created by the author based on data found in endnote 10

12   Mayo Clinic Staff, Mayo Clinic, Healthy Lifestyle, Nutrition and Healthy Eating, "Chart of High Fiber Foods" accessed November 5, 2919, https://www.mayoclinic.org/healthy-lifestyle/nutrition-and-healthy-eating/in-depth/high-fiber-foods/art-20050948.

13   Ellen G. White, "Chap. 4 - Relation of Diet to Health and Morals," *Christian Temperance and Bible Hygiene 47* (1890)

14   Ellen G. White, "Chap. 23 – Diet and Health, Preparation of Food," *Ministry of Healing 300* (1905)

15   Figure 4 was created by the author based on United States Department of Agriculture, Agriculture Research Service, "A Look at Calorie Sources in the American Diet," accessed November 5, 2019, https://www.ers.usda.gov/amber-waves/2016/december/a-look-at-calorie-sources-in-the-american-diet/.

16   Michael D. Crowell et al., "Emerging Drugs for Chronic Constipation," *Expert Opinion on Emerging Drugs* 24 (2009): 493–504.

17   M. Katherine Hoy and Joseph D. Goldman, Food Surveys Research Group Dietary Data Brief No. 12, U.S. Department of Agriculture, Agricultural Research Service Fiber intake of the U.S. population "What We Eat in America, NHANES 2009-2010" accessed November 5, 2019, https://www.ars.usda.gov/ARSUserFiles/80400530/pdf/DBrief/12_fiber_intake_0910.pdf.

18   Dietary Guidelines for Americans 2015-2020 Eighth Edition, accessed on November 5, 2019, https://health.gov/dietaryguidelines/2015/guidelines/.

19   Physicians Committee for Responsible Medicine, "Fiber Fill Up on 40 Grams of Fiber a Day" accessed on November 5, 2019 https://www.pcrm.org/good-nutrition/nutrition-information/fiber

20   Figure 5 was created by the author based on data found in endnote 17.

21   A. Kuijsten, et.al, "Dietary Fibre and Incidence of Type 2 Diabetes in Eight European Countries: The EPIC-InterAct Study and a Meta-Analysis of Prospective Studies," *Diabetologia* 58, no. 7 (July 2015): 1394–1408.

22   Figure 6 was created by the author based on data found in USDA National Nutrient Database for Standard Reference, Release 27

23   Laurenmu, "Homemade Black Bean Veggie Burgers" accessed November 5, 2019 https://www.allrecipes.com/recipe/85452/

homemade-black-bean-veggie-burgers/?internalSource=hub%20
recipe&referringContentType=Search&clickId=cardslot%201

24 Maria Speck, "Almond-Honey Power Bar," EatingWell Magazine, January/
February 2010 accessed November 5, 2019 www.eatingwell.com/recipe/253052.

Chapter 10. What to Drink?

1   USGS, "The Water in You: Water and the Human Body" accessed November 5,
2019, https://www.usgs.gov/special-topic/water-science-school/science/water-
you-water-and-human-body?qt-science_center_objects=0#qt-science_center_
objects

2   Michael. J. Orlich et al., "Patterns of Food Consumption among Vegetarians
and Non-Vegetarians," British Journal of Nutrition 112, no. 10 (November 2014):
1644–53.

3   Figure 1 was created by the author based on data found in reference 2.

4   Jacqueline Chan et al., "Water, Other Fluids, and Fatal Coronary Heart Disease:
The Adventist Health Study," American Journal of Epidemiolog, 155, no. 9 (2002):
827–33.

5   Figure 2 was created by the author based on data found in reference 4.

6   Ellen G. White, "Chap. 17 - The Use of Remedies," Ministry of Healing 237 (1905)

7   Figure 3 was created by the author based on data found in reference 4.

8   Dominique S. Michaud et al., "Fluid Intake and the Risk of Bladder Cancer in
Men," The New England Journal of Medicine 340, no. 18 (May 6, 1999): 1390–93.

9   Figure 4 was created by the author based on data found in reference 8.

10 Ameneh Madjid et al., "Effects on Weight Loss in Adults of Replacing Diet
Beverages with Water during a Hypoenergetic Diet: A Randomized, 24-Week
Clinical Trial," American Journal of Clinical Nutrition 101 (2015): 1305–12.

11 Helen M. Parretti et al., "Efficacy of Water Preloading before Main Meals as a
Strategy for Weight Loss in Primary Care Patients with Obesity: RCT," Obesity
23, no. 9 (September 2015): 1785–91.

12 Naiman A. Khan et al., "The Relationship between Total Water Intake and
Cognitive Control among Prepubertal Children," Annals of Nutrition &
Metabolism 66 Suppl 3 (2015): 38–41.

13 Clinton S. Perry et al., "Hydration Status Moderates the Effect of Drinking
Water on Children's Cognitive Performance, Appetite 95 (December 2015):
520–27.

14 Alice Callahan, "Is Alkaline Water Really Better for You?" New York Times
print edition page D4, accessed November 5, 2019, https://www.nytimes.
com/2018/04/27/well/eat/alkaline-water-health-benefits.html

15 Medical News Today, "What is alkaline water?," https://www.medicalnewstoday.com/articles/313681.php.

16 Michael. J. Orlich et al., "Patterns of Food Consumption among Vegetarians and Non-Vegetarians," *British Journal of Nutrition* 112, no. 10 (November 2014): 1644–53.

17 Figure 5 was created by the author based on data found in reference 16.

18 Ellen G. White, *Manuscript 126 1903*

19 Ellen G. White, *Letter 89a, 1894*, reprinted in *Vol. 6 Manuscript Releases 135*

20 Gitanjali Singh et al., "Estimated Global, Regional, and National Disease Burdens Related to Sugar-Sweetened Beverage Consumption in 2010," *Circulation* June 29, 2015: 115 pages.

21 Michael. J. Orlich et al., "Patterns of Food Consumption among Vegetarians and Non-Vegetarians," *British Journal of Nutrition* 112, no. 10 (November 2014): 1644–53.

22 Figure 6 was created by the author based on data found in reference 21.

23 M. Shahbandeh, Statista, "Domestic consumption of coffee in the United States from 2013/14 to 2018/19 (in million 60-kilogram bags)" accessed November 5, 2019, https://www.statista.com/statistics/804271/domestic-coffee-consumption-in-the-us/

24 Dan Bolton, "Insight: U.S. Organic Tea Imports," World Tea News, Feb 28, 2017, accessed November 5, 2019, https://worldteanews.com/tea-industry-news-and-features/insight-u-s-organic-tea-imports

25 Jan Conway, "Energy drink sales in the United States from 2015 to 2018 (in million U.S. dollars)" Statista accessed November 5, 2019, https://www.statista.com/statistics/558022/us-energy-drink-sales/.

26 Figure 7 was created by the author based on data found in reference 16.

27 Ming Ding et al., "Association of Coffee Consumption with Total and Cause-Specific Mortality in 3 Large Prospective Cohorts," *Circulation* 132, no. 24 (December 15, 2015): 2305–15.

28 Kristian Lindsted et al., "Coffee Consumption and Cause-Specific Mortality," *Journal of Clinical Epidemiology* 45, no. 7 (1992): 733–42.

29 Figure 8 was created by the author based on data found in reference 28.

30 Figure 9 was created by the author based on data found in reference 28.

31 Figure 10 was created by the author based on data found in reference 28.

32 Figure 11 was created by the author based on data found in reference 28.

33 Ellen G. White, "Tea and Coffee" Chapter – 26 Stimulants and Narcotics, *Ministry of Healing 326* (1905)

34 Figure 12 was created by the author based on data found in reference 21.

35 Daniel J. DeNoon, "How Much Caffeine Is in Your Energy Drink?" WebMD, Food & Recipes, October 25, 2012, accessed November 5, 2019, https://www.webmd.com/food-recipes/news/20121025/how-much-caffeine-energy-drink#2

36 Center for Science in the Public Interest, The Coffee Chart, accessed on November 5, 2019, https://cspinet.org/eating-healthy/ingredients-of-concern/caffeine-chart

Chapter 11. The Dairy Delema

1   C. Agostoni and D. J. Turck, "Is Cow's Milk Harmful to a Child's Health?" Journal of Pediatric Gastroenterology and Nutrition 53, no. 6 (December 2011): 594–600.

2   Michael J. Orlich et al., "Patterns of Food Consumption among Vegetarians and Non-Vegetarians," British Journal of Nutrition 112, no. 10 (November 2014): 1644–53.

3   Figure 1 was created by the author based on data found in reference 2.

4   Michael J. Orlich et al., "Patterns of Food Consumption among Vegetarians and Non-Vegetarians," British Journal of Nutrition 112, no. 10 (November 2014): 1644–53.

5   Figure 2 was created by the author based on data found in reference 4.

6   Michael J. Orlich et al., "Patterns of Food Consumption among Vegetarians and Non-Vegetarians," British Journal of Nutrition 112, no. 10 (November 2014): 1644–53.

7   Figure 3 was created by the author based on data found in reference 6.

8   Ellen G. White, "Chapter 5 – Extremes in Diet," Christian Temperance and Bible Hygiene 57

9   Centers for Disease Control and Prevention, CDC Features, "Raw (Unpasteurized) Milk," accessed November 11, 2019, https://www.cdc.gov/features/rawmilk/.

10 Ellen G. White, "Chapter 23-Diet and Health," Ministry of Healing 302 (1905)

11 Ellen G. White, "Chapter 21-Fats," Letter 39, 1901 republished in Counsels on Diet and Food 357.

12 Ellen G. White, "Section 4-The Health Work," Vol. 9 Testimonies for the Church 162 (1909)

13 Karl Michaelsson et al., "Milk Intake and Risk of Mortality and Fractures in Women and Men: Cohort Studies," British Medical Journal October 27, 2014: 1-15.

14 Figure 4 was created by the author based on data found in reference 13 table F.

15 Figure 5 was created by the author based on data from reference 13 Table F.

16 Figure 6 was created by the author based on data from reference 13 Table F.

17 Thomas Campbell, MD, "12 Frightening Facts about Milk," October 31, 2014, accessed November 11, 2019 https://nutritionstudies.org/?s=milk.

18 Figure 7 was created by the author based on data found in U.S. Department of Agriculture, Agricultural Research Service. FoodData Central, 2019 accessed on November 11, 2019.

19 Figure 8 "Trends in U.S. Per Capita Consumption of Dairy Products, 1970-2012" This article is drawn from...*Food Availability (Per Capita) Data System,* by Jeanine Bentley and Linda Kantor, USDA, Economic Research Service, August 2019 accessed November 11, 2019 https://www.ers.usda.gov/amber-waves/2014/june/trends-in-us-per-capita-consumption-of-dairy-products-1970-2012/.

20 https://en.wikipedia.org/wiki/Cheese, accessed November 11, 2019.

21 Ibid

22 M. Shahbandeh, "Per capita consumption of cheese in the United States from 2000 to 2018 (in pounds)," Statista, last edited Sep 17, 2019 accessed November 19, 2019, https://www.statista.com/statistics/183785/per-capita-consumption-of-cheese-in-the-us-since-2000/

23 Figure 9 was created by the author based on data found in reference 6.

24 Paul K. Mills et al., "Dietary Habits and Breast Cancer Incidence among Seventh-day Adventists," *Cancer* 64 (1989): 582–90.

25 Figure 10 was created by the author based on data found in reference 24.

26 Fatemeh Kiani et al., "Dietary Risk Factors for Ovarian Cancer: The Adventist Health Study (United States)," *Cancer Causes and Control* 17 (2006): 137–46.

27 Figure 11 was created by the author based on data found in reference 26.

28 Ellen G. White, "Chap. 4 - Relation of Diet to Health and Morals," *Christian Temperance and Bible Hygiene 46*, (1890)

29 Ellen G. White, "Chap. 7 - Neglect of Health Reform," Vol. 2 Testimonies for the Church 68 (1868-1871)

30 Ellen G. White, "Letter 1, 1873" reprinted in Chapter-22 Protein, Counsels on Diet and Food. (1938)

31 M. Shahbandeh, "Per capita consumption of butter in the United States from 2000 to 2018 (in pounds)*" Statista accessed November 11, 2019. https://www.statista.com/statistics/184011/per-capita-consumption-of-butter-in-the-us-since-2000/.

32 The Data Team, "Margarine sales: investors can't believe they're not better" *The Economist, Apr 17th 2017* accessed November 19,2019. https://www.economist.com/graphic-detail/2017/04/17/margarine-sales-investors-cant-believe-theyre-not-better.

33 Ellen G. White, "Chapter 23-Diet and Health" *Ministry of Healing 302* (1905)

34 Ellen G. White, "Section 14, Teaching Health Principles," *Letter 331 1904* reprinted in *Medical Ministry 269* (1932)

35 Ellen G. White, "Chapter 23-Diet and Health." *Ministry of Healing 298* (1905)

36 Figure 12 was created by the author based on data found in reference 6.

37 Figure 13 was created by the author based on data found in reference 6.

38   Nonsikelelo Mathe et al., "Dietary Patterns in Adults with Type 2 Diabetes Predict Cardiometabolic Risk Factors," *Canadian Journal of Diabetes* 40 (August 2016): 296–303.

39   A. Talaie-Zaniani et al., "A Comparative Study of Nutritional Status and Foodstuffs in Adolescent Girls in Iran," *Annals of Medical Health Scientific Reviews* 4, no. 1 (January–February 2014): 38–43.

40   Atsumi Hamada et al., "Deterioration of Traditional Dietary Custom Increases the Risk of Lifestyle-Related Diseases in Young Male Africans," *Journal of Biomedical Science* 17 Suppl 1 (2010): S34 6 pages.

41   William K. Bosu, "An Overview of the Nutritional Transition in West Africa: Implications for Non-Communicable Diseases," *Proceedings of Nutritional Society* 74, no. 4 (November 2015): 466–77.

42   Ellen G. White, "Chapter 19-Desserts," *Manuscript 87, 1908* reprinted in Counsels on Diet and Foods (1938)

43   A. Tavani et al., "Consumption of Sweet Foods and Breast Cancer Risk in Italy," *Annals of Oncology* 17, no. 2 (February 2006): 341–45.

44   M. T. Goodman et al., "High-fat Foods and the Risk of Lung Cancer," *Epidemiology* 3, no. 4 (July 1992): 288–99.

45   Janet L. Colli and Albert Colli, "Comparisons of Prostate Cancer Mortality Rates with Dietary Practices in the United States," *Urology Oncology* 23, no. 6 (November–December 2005): 390–98.

46   Georgina E. Crichton et al., "Dairy Intake and Cognitive Health in Middle-Aged South Australians," *Asia Pacific Journal of Clinical Nutrition* 19, no. 2 (2010): 161–71.

47   U.S. Department of Agriculture "Choose My Plate," the *Dietary Guidelines for Americans 2015-2020*, accessed November 11, 2019, https://www.choosemyplate.gov/2015-2020-dietary-guidelines-answers-your-questions.

48   United States Department of Agriculture, Agriculture Research Service, Food Data Central Search Results accessed November 11, 2019, https://fdc.nal.usda.gov/fdc-app.html#/food-details/171287/nutrients

49   Michael J. Orlich et al., "Patterns of Food Consumption among Vegetarians and Non-Vegetarians," *British Journal of Nutrition* 112, no. 10 (November 2014): 1644–53.

50   Figure 14 was created by the author based on data found in reference 49.

51   Victor W. Zhong et al., "Associations of Dietary Cholesterol or Egg Consumption with Incident Cardiovascular Disease and Mortality," *Journal of the American Medical Association* 321, no. 11 (March 19, 2019): 1081–95.

52   Figure 15 was created by the author based on data found in reference 51.

53   Figure 16 was created by the author based on data found in reference 51

54   Ellen G. White, "Faithfulness in Health Reform," *Counsels to the Church 237*

55   Ellen G. White, "Chapter 11-Extremes in Diet," Letter 37, 1905 reprinted in *Counsels on Diet and Health 206* (1938)

Chapter 12. Preferable Protein for a Healthy Diet

1   Ellen G. White, "Chapter XIV-Causes of Diseases," Healthful Living 67 (1897)

2   Ellen G. White, "Flesh as Food," *Ministry of Healing 315* (1905)

3   Michael. J. Orlich et al., "Patterns of Food Consumption among Vegetarians and Non-Vegetarians," *British Journal of Nutrition* 112, no. 10 (November 2014): 1644–53.

4   Figure 1 was created by the author based on data found in reference 3.

5   David A. Snowdon et al., "Meat Consumption and Fatal Ischemic Heart Disease," *Preventive Medicine* 13 (1984): 490–500.

6   Figure 2 was created by the author based on data found in reference 5.

7   Marioin Tharrey et al., "Patterns of Plant and Animal Protein Intake Are Strongly Associated with Cardiovascular Mortality: The Adventist Health Study-2 Cohort," *International Journal of Epidemiology* April 2, 2018: 1603–12.

8   Figure 3 was created by the author based on data found in reference 7.

9   Figure 4 was created by the author based on data found in reference 7.

10   Rebecca L. Siegel et al., "Cancer Statistics 2017," *CA A Cancer Journal for Clinicians*, 67, no. 1 (January/February 2017): 7–30.

11   Pramil N. Singh and Gary E. Fraser, "Dietary Risk Factors for Colon Cancer in a Low-risk Population," *American Journal of Epidemiology* 148, no. 8 (1998): 761–74.

12   Figure 5 was created by the author based on data found in reference 11.

13   Paul K. Mills et al., "Dietary Habits and Past Medical History as Related to Fatal Pancreas Cancer Risk among Adventists," *Cancer* 61 (1988): 2578–85.

14   Figure 6 was created by the author based on data found in reference 13.

15   Rebecca L. Siegel et al., "Cancer Statistics 2017," *CA A Cancer Journal for Clinicians*, 67, no. 1 (January/February 2017): 7–30.

16   Paul K. Mills et al., "Bladder Cancer in a Low Risk Population: Results from the Adventist Health Study," *American Journal of Epidemiology* 133, no. 3 (February 1991): 230–39.

17   Figure 7 was created by the author based on data found in reference 16.

18   Rebecca L. Siegel et al., "Cancer Statistics 2017," *CA A Cancer Journal for Clinicians*, 67, no. 1 (January/February 2017): 7–30.

19   Fatima Kiani et al., "Dietary Risk Factors for Ovarian Cancer: The Adventist Health Study," *Cancer Causes and Control* 17 (2006): 137–46.

20   Figure 8 was created by the author based on data found in reference 19.

21   Gary E. Fraser, "Vegetarian Diets: What Do We Know of Their Effects on Common Chronic Diseases?" *American Journal of Clinical Nutrition* 89 (2009): 1607S-1612S.

22   Figure 9 was created by the author based on data found in reference 21.

23   Paul L. Huang, "A comprehensive definition for metabolic syndrome," Disease Models and Mechanisms, 2009 May-Jun; 2(5-6): 231–237.

24   Nico S. Rizzo et al., "Vegetarian Dietary Patterns Are Associated with a Lower Risk of Metabolic Syndrome: The Adventist Health Study 2," *Diabetes Care* 34, no. 5 (May 2011): 1225–27.

25   Rashmi Sinha et al., "Meat Intake and Mortality: A Prospective Study of Over Half a Million People," *Archives of Internal Medicine* 169, no. 6 (March 23, 2009): 562–71.

26   Figure 10 was created by the author based on data found in reference 25.

27   Figure 11 was created by the author based on data found in reference 25.

28   Rachael. Z. Stolzenberg-Solomon et al., "Meat and Meat-Mutagen Intake and Pancreatic Cancer Risk in the NIH-AARP Cohort," *Cancer Epidemiology Biomarkers and Prevention* 16, no. 12 (December 2007): 2664–75.

29   Amanda J. Cross et al., "A Prospective Study of Red and Processed Meat Intake in Relation to Cancer Risk," *PLOS Medicine* 4, no. 12 (December 2007): 1973–76.

Chapter 13. Other Healthful Lifestyle Factors Beyond Diet

1   Ellen G. White, "Chapter 8-The Physician, an Educator," Ministry of Healing 127, (1905)

2   Stacy Simon, "World Health Organization: Outdoor Air Pollution Causes Cancer," American Cancer Society News, accessed November 12,2019 https://www.cancer.org/latest-news/world-health-organization-outdoor-air-pollution-causes-cancer.html

3   Robyn. Lucas et al., "Solar Ultraviolet Radiation: Global Burden of Disease from Solar Ultraviolet Radiation," *Environmental Burden of Disease Series* no. 13 (2006), 258 pages.

4   M. Nathaniel Mead, "Benefits of Sunlight: A Bright Spot for Human Health," *Environmental Health Perspectives*. 2008 Apr; 116(4): A160–A167.

5   National Institutes of Health, Department of Health and Human Services, newsinhealth.nih.gov, "The Benefits of Slumber, Why You Need a Good Night's Sleep" April 2013, accessed November 12, 2019, https://newsinhealth.nih.gov/sites/nihNIH/files/2013/April/NIHNiHApr2013.pdf

6   Jean-Philippe Chaput, et.al, "Sleeping hours: what is the ideal number and how does age impact this?" *Nature and Science of Sleep* 2018:10 421–430.

7   Figure 1 is a table which was created by the author based on data found in reference 6.

8   U.S. Department of Health and Human Services, Physical Activity Guidelines for Americans second edition, 2018 accessed November 12, 2019, https://health.gov/paguidelines/second edition/pdf/Physical_Activity_Guide-lines_2nd_edition.pdf#page=55.

9   Ellen G. White, "Chapter 2-Exercise and Air, *Vol 2, Testimonies for the Church 525.* (1868-1871)

10 Ellen G. White, "Chapter 17-The use of Remedies," *Ministry of Healing 237.*

11 Harold G. Koenig, *The Healing Power of Faith: How Belief and Prayer Can Help You Triumph over Diseases* (United States of America: Touchstone, 2001).

12 Kelly R. Morton et al., "Pathways from Religion to Health: Mediation by Psychosocial and Lifestyle Mechanisms," *Psychology of Religion and Spirituality* 9, no. 1 (February 2017): 108–17.

Chapter 14. What the Healthiest People Avoid

1   The Oxford Dictionary of Phrase and Fable, "Moderation in all Things" Updated October 4, 2019. Accessed November 11, 2019, https://www.encyclopedia.com/humanities/dictionaries-thesauruses-pictures-and-press-releases/moderation-all-things.

2   World Health Organization, Tobacco, NMH Fact Sheet June 2009, accessed November 11, 2019, https://www.who.int/nmh/publications/fact_sheet_tobacco_en.pdf

3   National Cancer Institute, About Cancer, Cancer Causes and Prevention, Tobacco, accessed November 12, 2019, https://www.cancer.gov/about-cancer/causes-prevention/risk/tobacco

4   Center for Disease Control and Prevention, Smoking and Tobacco use, "Heart Disease and Strokes," accessed November 12, 2019, https://www.cdc.gov/tobacco/basic_information/health_effects/heart_disease/index.htm

5   Johns Hopkins Medicine, Health, Conditions and Diseases, "Smoking and Respiratory Diseases" accessed November 13 2019, https://www.hopkinsmedicine.org/health/conditions-and-diseases/smoking-and-respiratory-diseases.

6   Ellen G. White, "Chapter XXXIX-Health," *Spiritual Gifts, vol. 4a, p. 128 (1864).*

7   Michael Orlich et al., "Vegetarian Dietary Patterns and Mortality in Adventist Health Study 2," *Journal of the American Medical Association (JAMA) Internal Medicine* 173, no. 13 (July 8, 2013): 1230–38.

8   Figure 1 was created by the author based on data found in reference 7.

9   Ellen G. White, Section Two-Our Sanitarium Work' "A Message to Our Physicians," *Volume 7, Testimonies for the Church 75.*

10 Figure 2 was created by the author based on data found in reference 7.

11 Figure 3 was created by the author based on data found in reference 7.

12 Judith Grisel, "One Salient Example: THC," in *Never Enough* (New York: Knopf Doubleday Publishing Group, Kindle Edition, 2019), 50-61.

13 Edmund Silins et al., "Young Adult Sequelae of Adolescent Cannabis Use: An Integrative Analysis," *Lancet Psychiatry* 1 (September 2014): 286–93.

14 Figure 4 was created by the author based on data found in reference 13.

15 Marta Di-Forte et al., "The Contribution of Cannabis Use to Variation in the Incidence of Psychotic Disorder across Europe" (EU_GEI): A Multicenter Case-Control Study, *Lancet Psychiatry* (March 19, 2019): 9 pages.

16 Figure 5 was created by the author based on data found in reference 15.

17 Edmund Silins et al., "Young Adult Sequelae of Adolescent Cannabis Use: An Integrative Analysis," *Lancet Psychiatry* 1 (September 2014): 286–93.

18 Figure 6 was created by the author based on data found in reference 17.

19 National Institute of Mental Health, Mental Health Information, "Suicide," accessed November 13, 2019, https://www.nimh.nih.gov/health/statistics/suicide.shtml.

20 Edmund Silins et al., "Young Adult Sequelae of Adolescent Cannabis Use: An Integrative Analysis," *Lancet Psychiatry* 1 (September 2014): 286–93.

21 Figure 7 was created by the author based on data found in reference 20.

22 Zachary Lipsman, MD, PGY2, Brown University, Emergency Medicine Residency, "A High Potency Opioid: Carfentanil, Lethal and on the Rise" American College of Emergency Physicians, Toxicology Section, accessed November 13, 2019. https://www.acep.org/how-we-serve/sections/toxicology/news/april-2017/a-high-potency-opioid-carfentanil-lethal-and-on-the-rise/

Chapter 15. Practicing a Healthful Lifestyle

1 George W. Comstock and K. B. Partridge, "Church Attendance and Health," *Journal of Chronic Diseases* 25 (1972): 665–72.

2 Marino A. Bruce et al., "Church Attendance, Allostatic Load and Mortality in Middle Aged Adults," *Plos One* 12, no. 5 (May 16, 2017) 1-14.

3 Earl S. Ford et al., "Healthy Living Is the Best Revenge: Findings from the European Prospective Investigation into Cancer and Nutrition-Potsdam Study," *Archives of Internal Medicine* 169, no. 15 (August 10/24, 2009): 1355–62.

4 Figure 1 was created by the author based on data found in reference 3.

5 Figure 2 was created by the author based on data found in reference 3.

6 Figure 3 was created by the author based on data found in reference 3.

7 Figure 4 was created by the author based on data found in reference 3.

APPENDIX A

How to Read Scientific Graphs

There are many graphs displaying scientific information on almost every page in this book. The main style of graph is the simple two-axis bar graph. If you understand the design elements used in these graphs, you can quickly grasp the point being made.

The most common graph is a vertical bar graph. The title appears at the top and will present the disease and the variable being examined. A disease might be colon cancer, and the variable might be citrus fruit. Often the size of the study population in the analysis will be included in the title.

In all the graphs, we are dealing with death or disease ratios. Ratios are easier to understand than rates or raw numbers. The columns display the dose or amount of a variable. The lowest dose is always on the left. The lowest dose is the reference point, the people who do the behavior the least. The highest dose is always on the right. These people did the behavior the most. These people ate a food item most or did the most exercise. Columns in the middle represent people with intermediate levels of practice.

So if we were looking at colon cancer deaths as related to citrus fruit in the diet, the people who used no citrus would be represented in the left column. Those with the highest use of citrus would be on the right. The dose in each category is listed at the bottom of each column.

For ease of comparison, the amount of disease, the death rate, the sickness rate, or the number of the lowest user of some variable is always adjusted to be one. In the columns to the right, if the columns get shorter and shorter, there is an advantage in reduced death rates or sickness with the increasing amount of a specific food.

In the sample graph below, notice that the middle dose experienced a death rate that was 0.7 compared with those with the lowest dose. This translates into a 30 percent reduction in the risk of death to those using the middle dose. Those with the highest dose had a death rate of 0.4 compared to those with the lowest dose. This translates into a 60 percent reduction in death.

In the graphs presented throughout this book, the brackets and percent advantage are not presented but simply the ratio. The percent advantage is presented in the text.

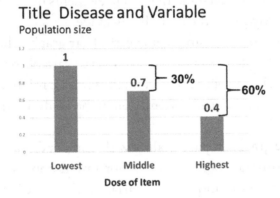

In some graphs, the bars go up with increasing dose. Increasing bar length indicates things going bad with increasing dose. An example would be cigarette smoking and lung cancer.

For example, the death rate from lung cancer for nonsmokers would be made one. The lowest dose is in the bar at the left side of the graph. As the dose of smoking increases, the risk of lung cancer increases. If the mortality ratio for the middle dose was 1.8, that would represent an 80 percent increase above the rate of nonsmokers.

When the highest dose is reached, the mortality ratio is now 2.4, which represents a 140 percent increase over nonsmokers. (The ratio is about twenty-seven times higher for the smokers of the highest number of cigarettes.) The point is, the increase is *not* 240 percent since the ratio is 2.4. The number 2.4 is only 1.4 times higher than the baseline of 1. The increase is only 140 percent.

The title of each graph is labeled a *Figure*, with a number indicating the sequence of that figure in the chapter. There will also be a brief description of what is being displayed in the graph. The scientific validity of the results displayed in the graph is measured by statistical probability, designated by *Significance p =*. In scientific research there is universal agreement that for an association or correlation of occurrence to be considered valid, it must have a less than 5 percent chance of being accidental or coincidental.

A statistically significant p value is 0.05 or smaller. Often the p value is extremely small, perhaps 0.001, which would indicate there is only one chance in 1,000 that the occurrence was accidental. The smaller the p value, the more valid the observation. So if the p value is 0.4, there is a 40 percent likelihood that the correlation was due to chance. This is not an acceptable level of proof.

Another way of expressing this is by the 95 percent *confidence interval* or *CI*. In this method of measuring significance, the range of values on either side of the reported value are displayed, showing the variability that exists at the 95 percent confidence interval. The wider the CI, the less stable is the reported number.

Title Disease and Variable
Population size

211

The sources for information in the text and graphs will be referenced by a small superscript number. The full reference is found in the endnotes at the back of the book.

Throughout this book the graphs do not have brackets or the percentages you see in this sample graph—just the ratios. The percentage expressing the advantage or disadvantage is important to understand and can be calculated from the ratios presented.

APPENDIX B

Glossary of Scientific Terms

AHS: Adventist Health Study (see appendix C).

all-cause mortality: A term used by epidemiologists, or disease-tracking scientists, to refer to death from all causes combined.

amino acids: The basic building blocks from which proteins are formed. Of the twenty amino acids used to construct human proteins, ten are "essential" amino acids that must be in the diet. The other amino acids can be synthesized within the human body.

antigen: A toxin, virus, bacteria, or other foreign substance that induces an immune response in the body, especially the production of antibodies.

antioxidant: A substance that inhibits oxidation (deterioration and breakdown), especially one used to counteract the deterioration of stored food product.

blinded study: A study done so the patients or subjects do not know (are blinded as to) what treatment they are receiving, to ensure that the results are not affected by a placebo effect (the power of suggestion). (Also see double-blind study below.)

BMI (body mass index): A weight-to-height ratio, calculated by dividing one's weight in kilograms by the square of one's height in meters and used as an indicator of obesity and overweight.

Normal	BMI 18.0–24.9
Overweight	BMI 25–29.9
Obesity	BMI 30+

Bragg Liquid Aminos: Bragg is a brand name of liquid aminos made from non-GMO soybeans and purified water. They are a replacement for tamari and soy sauce. Liquid aminos are not fermented or heated and are gluten-free.

C-reactive protein (CRP): One of the plasma proteins known as acute-phase proteins: proteins whose plasma concentrations increase (or decrease) by 25 percent or more during inflammatory disorders. CRP can rise as high as a thousand fold with inflammation. Conditions that commonly lead to marked changes in CRP include infection, trauma, surgery, burns, inflammatory conditions, and advanced cancer. Moderate changes occur after strenuous exercise, heatstroke, and childbirth. Small changes occur after psychological stress and in several psychiatric illnesses.

cholesterol: A compound of the sterol type found in most body tissues. Cholesterol and its derivatives are important constituents of cell membranes and precursors of other steroid compounds, but a high proportion in the blood of low-density lipoprotein (LDL), which transports cholesterol from the liver to the tissues, is associated with an increased risk of coronary heart disease.

CI (confidence interval): A range of values defined so there is a specified probability that the value of a parameter lies within it. Usually the interval is defined so there is a 95 percent probability that the "true" value lies between the upper and lower value of the interval.

cis fatty acid: A natural fatty acid, in which the hydrogen atoms attached to a carbon molecule lie on the same side of a double bond. In nature, fats and oils contain only cis double bonds. A cis double bond causes a sharp bend in the fatty acid that makes these fats more liquid. In heating and hydrogenating cis fatty acids, they frequently transform to *trans* configurations, which straighten up the fatty acids and makes them appear and perform like saturated fatty acids. (See trans-fatty acid below.)

confidence limits: The highest and lowest values of a confidence interval.

cruciferous vegetables: Vegetables of the family Brassicaceae (also called Cruciferae), with many genera, species, and cultivars being raised for food production, such as cauliflower, cabbage, garden cress, bok choy, broccoli, brussels sprouts, and similar green leafy vegetables.

diglyceride: A glycerol molecule with two fatty acids attached. (Also see monoglyceride and triglyceride below.)

double-blind study: A double-blind study is one in which neither the participants nor the experimenters know who is receiving a particular treatment. This procedure is utilized to prevent bias in research results. Double-blind studies are useful for preventing bias due to patient expectations or researcher prejudice. (Also see blinded study above.)

epidemiology: The branch of medicine that deals with the distribution of disease in a population. It includes the possible control of diseases and other factors relating to health.

experimental studies: Ones where researchers introduce an intervention and study the effects. Experimental studies are usually randomized, meaning eligible people are randomly assigned to one of two or more groups. One group receives the intervention (such as a new drug), while the other, the control group, receives nothing or an inactive placebo. The researchers then study what happens to people in each group. Any difference in outcomes can then be linked to the intervention.

fiber, soluble and insoluble: Fiber (the portion of plants that cannot be digested by the human digestive tract) is classified as soluble or insoluble. Oats, beans, dried peas, and legumes are major sources of soluble fiber, whereas wheat bran, whole-grain products, and vegetables are major sources of insoluble fiber.

free radicals: Unstable atoms that can damage cells, causing illness and aging.

ghrelin: A hormone produced and released mainly by the stomach, with small amounts also released by the small intestine, pancreas, and brain. Ghrelin has numerous functions. It is termed the "hunger hormone" because it stimulates appetite, increases food intake, and promotes fat storage. When administered to humans, ghrelin increases food intake by up to 30 percent.

glycemic index: A number that shows you about how fast your body converts the carbohydrates in a food into glucose. Two foods with the same amount of carbohydrates can have different glycemic index numbers. The smaller the glycemic index number, the less impact the food has on your blood sugar.

- 55 or less = Low (good)
- 56– 69 = Medium
- 70 or higher = High (bad)

GMO: A genetically modified organism results from a laboratory process where genes from the DNA of one species are extracted and inserted into the DNA of an unrelated plant or animal.

Gram: A metric unit of mass equal to one thousandth of a kilogram. It is 0.035 of an ounce.

gut microbiome: The human microbiome comprises trillions of organisms, including bacteria, viruses, and fungi. The biggest populations of microbes reside in the colon.

HDL cholesterol: High density lipoprotein cholesterol. Lipoproteins, which are combinations of fats (lipids) and proteins, are the form in which lipids are transported in the blood. An HDL cholesterol of 60 mg/dL or higher gives some protection against heart disease.

hypertension: High blood pressure. Blood pressure is expressed in two numbers, a higher (systolic) over the lower (diastolic). The two numbers describe the range of pressure in your major arteries that occurs from heartbeat to heartbeat.

immune system: The bodily system that protects the body from foreign substances, cells, and tissues by producing the immune response. It includes especially the thymus, spleen, lymph nodes, special deposits of lymphoid tissue (as in the gastrointestinal tract and bone marrow), macrophages, lymphocytes including the B cells and T cells, and antibodies.

interleukin 6 (IL-6): One of a large group of interleukins. Interleukins are circulating blood proteins that send signals among various cells of the body. They are made by white blood cells and some other cells. Interleukin-6 is made mainly by some T lymphocytes, which are a white blood cell that matures in the thymus gland in the chest. IL-6 promotes inflammation by causing B lymphocytes, which are a white blood cell that matures in bone marrow, to make more antibodies and causes fever by affecting areas of the brain that control body temperature.

LDL cholesterol: Low-density lipoprotein cholesterol, commonly called "bad" cholesterol. Elevated LDL levels are associated with an increased risk of heart disease. Lipoproteins are combinations of fats (lipids) and proteins and are the form in which cholesterol and fats are transported in the blood. Low-density lipoproteins transport cholesterol from the liver to the tissues of the body.

legumes: Legumes come from the family of plants called Leguminosae. A trait all legumes share is that they grow in a pod. Legumes are high in protein and have a low-fat content, so they are generally considered healthy.

life expectancy: Refers to the number of years a person can expect to live. Life expectancy is based on an estimate of the average age that members of a population group will be when they die. Life expectancy is one of the key measures of a population's health and an indicator used widely by policy makers and researchers to complement economic measures of prosperity.

longevity: Longevity means long life. The word *longevity* is sometimes used as a synonym for life expectancy. Longevity is sometimes meant to refer only to especially long-lived members of a population, whereas life expectancy is always defined statistically as the average number of years remaining at a given age. Longevity is best thought of as a term for general audiences meaning typical length of life.

mean: The mean is the average of a set of numbers, a calculated "central" value of a set of numbers. It is derived by adding up all the numbers and then dividing by how many numbers there are in the set.

median: The median denotes or relates to a value or quantity lying at the midpoint of a frequency distribution of observed values or quantities, so there is an equal probability of falling above or below it.

metabolic syndrome: The name for a group of risk factors that raises your risk for heart disease, diabetes, and stroke. The five conditions described below are metabolic risk factors. You must have at least three metabolic risk factors to be diagnosed with metabolic syndrome.

1. A large waistline.

2. A high triglyceride level or you're on medicine to treat high triglycerides.
3. A low HDL cholesterol level or you're on medicine to treat low HDL cholesterol.
4. High blood pressure or you're on medicine to treat high blood pressure.
5. High fasting blood sugar or you're on medicine to treat high blood sugar.

monoglyceride: A glycerin molecule that has only one fatty acid attached. (Also see diglyceride and triglyceride.)

monounsaturated: Containing one double bond per molecule—especially of an oil, fat, or fatty acid.

mortality rates:
 total mortality: Measures all causes of death or overall mortality.
 crude mortality rate: The mortality rate from all causes of death for a population.
 cause-specific mortality rate: The mortality rate from a specified cause for a population.
 age-specific mortality rate: A mortality rate limited to a particular age group.

observational studies: Population studies in which individuals are observed or certain outcomes are measured. No attempt is made to affect the outcome—for example, no treatment is given.
 case-control study or retrospective study: A study originally developed in epidemiology, in which two existing groups differing in outcome are identified and compared based on some possible causal attribute. This type of study is useful when studying relatively rare diseases or conditions.
 cross-sectional study: Involves data collection from a population, or a representative subset, at one specific point in time.

longitudinal study or prospective study: Correlational research study that involves repeated observations of the same variables in the same population over long periods of time.

cohort study or panel study: A particular form of longitudinal study where a group of patients is closely monitored over time.

ounce: A unit of mass, weight, or volume used in most British-derived customary systems of measurement. An ounce is one-sixteenth of a pound, which is 28.35 grams.

overall mortality: Measures all causes of death combined. It is the same as all-cause mortality and total mortality.

oxidation: A process in which a chemical substance changes because of adding oxygen.

OXM (oxyntomodulin): A naturally occurring thirty-seven-amino acid peptide hormone found in the colon. It has been found to suppress appetite.

pesco-vegetarian: A vegetarian who includes fish in the diet and may include dairy products and eggs in addition to plant foods.

phytochemicals: Chemicals produced by plants in their growth and development. Because tens of thousands of these chemical compounds have just been recently discovered, the role of most of these phytochemicals in human health has not been established yet.

polyunsaturated: Means a fat or oil molecule containing several double bonds between carbon atoms. Polyunsaturated fats, which are usually of plant origin, are regarded as healthier in the diet than saturated fats.

prebiotic: A nondigestible fiber that promotes the growth of beneficial microorganisms in the intestines. Prebiotic fiber is naturally found in virtually all plant-based foods. Highly refined and often single fiber sources are sold as stand-alone supplements or are mixed with low-fiber foods in an attempt to enhance the health benefits of manufactured foods. (Also see synbiotics below.)

probability: The chance that something will happen; how likely it is that some event will occur.

probiotics: Commercially available supplements or foods that contain live bacteria and yeasts that are known to not cause disease and thus are potentially good for you, especially your digestive system. Usually, only a few species of organisms are included. There are many thousands of helpful organisms in the colon of healthy individuals. The value of commercially available probiotics has not been established. (Also see synbiotics below.)

prospective study: See observational studies above.

PYY (peptide tyrosine tyrosine): Hormones released from intestinal cells in response to a meal. These circulating hormones are satiety (satisfaction) signals, as they have been found to decrease food intake and body weight.

quartile: A statistical term describing a division of observations into four defined intervals based upon the values of the data and how they compare to the entire set of observations.

quintile: Any of five equal groups into which a population can be divided according to the distribution of values of a variable.

randomized: A study in which the participants are divided by chance into separate groups that compare different treatments or other interventions. Using chance to divide people into groups means that the groups will be similar and that the effects of the treatments they receive can be compared more fairly. At the time of the trial, it is not known which treatment is best.

retrospective study: See observational studies above.

saturated: An organic molecule (often a fatty acid) containing the greatest possible number of hydrogen atoms and so having no carbon-carbon double or triple bonds. These fats contribute to hardening of the arteries and cardiovascular diseases.

soluble fiber: See fiber above.

standardized mortality ratio: The standardized mortality ratio, or SMR, is a quantity expressed as either a ratio or percentage quantifying the increase or decrease in mortality of a study cohort with respect to the general population or reference group.

statistical significance: Refers to the claim that a result from data generated by testing or experimentation is not likely to occur randomly or by chance but is instead likely to be attributable to a specific cause.

synbiotics: Food ingredients or dietary supplements combining probiotics and prebiotics in a form of supposed synergism, hence synbiotics. (Also see prebiotics and probiotics above.)

tertile: A statistical term describing a division of observations into three defined intervals.

tissue necrosis factor-α (TNF): A cell-signaling protein involved in systemic inflammation. The primary role of TNF is in regulating immune cells. TNF can induce fever, cell death, and inflammation to inhibit the formation of cancers, and the propagation of viruses. When out of control, TNF affects several human diseases, including Alzheimer's disease, several cancers, major depression, psoriasis, and inflammatory bowel disease.

total mortality: See mortality rates above.

trans-fatty acid: An unsaturated fatty acid of a type occurring in hard margarines and manufactured cooking oils because of the hydrogenation process, having a *trans* arrangement (as opposed to a *cis* arrangement) of the carbon atoms adjacent to its double bonds. In a *trans* configuration of a double bond, the hydrogen molecules are on opposite sides of adjacent carbon atoms. This configuration makes an unsaturated fatty acid similar in configuration to a saturated fat. Consumption of such acids increases the risk of atherosclerosis. (Also see cis fatty acid above.)

triglyceride: Formed from glycerol and three fatty acid groups. Triglycerides are the main constituents of natural fats and oils, and high concentrations in the blood indicate an elevated risk of stroke.

unsaturated fats: Having carbon-carbon double bonds and therefore not containing the greatest possible number of hydrogen atoms for the number of carbons. These are considered the preferable fats for disease prevention.

variable: Any characteristic, number, or quantity that can be measured or counted.

vegan: A person who does not eat animal products, including eggs and dairy products, and whose diet consists entirely of plant-based foods.

vegetarian: A person who does not eat meat for moral, religious, or health reasons. A **lacto-ovo vegetarian** includes milk and eggs in an otherwise plant-based diet. A **strict vegetarian** is a vegan. A **pesco-vegetarian** includes fish and dairy products in an otherwise plant-based diet.

vital wheat gluten: Produced by several commercial flour mills. It is extracted from wheat flour and is the protein portion of the wheat. It can be used alone to make high-protein foods or added to other flours to produce a rising effect, making the flour lighter.

APPENDIX C

A Brief History of the Adventist Health Studies

Seventh-day Adventists have been the subject of several large epidemiologic studies over the past seventy years. Details regarding these studies, outlined below, are available at https://publichealth.llu.edu/adventist-health-studies/.

Adventist Mortality Study: This study was conducted from 1958 to 1966 and included twenty-three thousand California Adventists ages twenty-five and older. This study was conducted with the American Cancer Society study of non-Adventists. Comparisons were made for many causes of death between the two populations.

Adventist Health Study-1: This study was conducted from 1974 to 1988 and included 34,192 California Adventists ages twenty-five and older. This study investigated factors relating to the incidence of disease and mainly compared the different health habits, especially differences in diet, among different Adventists.

Adventist Health Air Pollution Study: This is an ongoing study started in 1976. It includes 6,328 California Adventists ages twenty-five and older. This is a substudy of Adventist Health Study-1 and was funded by the Environmental Protection Agency. Its goal is to link the effects of various indoor and outdoor pollutants with respiratory diseases and lung cancer.

Adventist Health Study-2 has been conducted from 2002 up to the present time. It is a study of ninety-six thousand Seventh-day Adventists in the United States and Canada. Adventists, due in part to their unique dietary habits, have a risk lower than other Americans of heart disease, several cancers, high blood pressure, arthritis, and diabetes. This, along with their wide variety of dietary habits, provides a special opportunity for careful research to answer a host of scientific questions about how diet (and other health habits) may change the risk of suffering from many chronic diseases.

Adventist Religion and Health Study: This study was initiated in 2006 and continues to the present time. It includes eleven thousand US and Canadian Adventists ages thirty and older. This is a substudy of Adventist Health Study-2, examining which aspects of religion account for better or worse health and tracing some of the bio-psycho-social pathways to health.

APPENDIX D

Ellen G. White Named among the Most Significant Americans

In the spring 2015 issue of *Smithsonian* magazine, Ellen G. White (November 26, 1827–July 16, 1915) was listed as one of the one hundred most significant Americans. She is listed along with the likes of Abraham Lincoln, Martin Luther King Jr., and Helen Keller.

Ellen White is the most widely published Seventh-day Adventist author. Her ministry spanned seventy years, from 1844 until 1915. Ellen White is credited as the cofounder of the Seventh-day Adventist Church. Guided by the Holy Spirit, Ellen White exalted Jesus and pointed to scripture as the basis of one's faith. She wrote on a wide variety of topics, from spirituality to health, education, ministry, and financial and marital advice.

Mrs. White wrote extensively on health throughout her lifetime. Scattered throughout the church's printed periodicals and books are many articles and chapters on various aspects of healthful living. After her death in 1915, her estate continued to compile health literature drawn from previous publications. All the writings of Ellen White, including all health books and articles, are accessible online at https://whiteestate.org/. Here is a listing of some books on health still available today. Those dated after 1915 are compilations assembled on health topics from the library of her writings by the staff of the E.G. White

Estate after her death. All these books are available online or at an Adventist Book Center.

Healthful Living (1897–1898)
Ministry of Healing (1905)
Counsels on Health (1923)
Medical Ministry (1932)
Counsels on Diets and Foods (1938)
Temperance (1949)
The Health Food Ministry (1970)
Mind, Character, and Personality, Volumes 1and 2 (1977)

APPENDIX E

Biblical References to Healthful Living

Here are a few selected texts on health issues from the New King James version of the Bible.

Texts on Health—A Gift from God

> Beloved, I pray that you may prosper in all things and be in health, just as your soul prospers. (3 John 1:2)

> Or do you not know that your body is the temple of the Holy Spirit who is in you, whom you have from God, and you are not your own? For you were bought at a price; therefore glorify God in your body and in your spirit, which are God's. (1 Corinthians 6:19–20)

> My son, give attention to my words; incline your ear to my sayings.
> Do not let them depart from your eyes; keep them in the midst of your heart;
> For they are life to those who find them, and health to all their flesh. (Proverbs 4:20–22)

Texts on Alcohol

> And do not be drunk with wine, in which is dissipation; but be filled with the Spirit. (Ephesians 5:18)

> Wine is a mocker, strong drink is a brawler, and whoever is led astray by it is not wise. (Proverbs 20:1)

> Do not mix with winebibbers, or with gluttonous eaters of meat; For the drunkard and the glutton will come to poverty, and drowsiness will clothe a man with rags. (Proverbs 23:20–21)

Texts on Clean and Unclean Flesh Foods

Clean and unclean animals for food was understood before the flood.

> Then the Lord said to Noah, "Come into the ark, you and all your household, because I have seen that you are righteous before Me in this generation. You shall take with you seven each of every clean animal, a male and his female; two each of animals that are unclean, a male and his female; (Genesis 7:1–2)

The original diet was liberalized after the flood.

> Every moving thing that lives shall be food for you. I have given you all things, even as the green herbs. But you shall not eat flesh with its life, that is, its blood. (Genesis 9:3–4)

Clean and unclean meats were defined.

> Now the Lord spoke to Moses and Aaron, saying to them, "Speak to the children of Israel, saying, "These

are the animals which you may eat among all the animals that are on the earth: Among the animals, whatever divides the hoof, having cloven hooves and chewing the cud—that you may eat. Nevertheless these you shall not eat among those that chew the cud or those that have cloven hooves: the camel, because it chews the cud but does not have cloven hooves, is unclean to you." (Leviticus 11:1–4)

To distinguish between the unclean and the clean, and between the animal that may be eaten and the animal that may not be eaten (Leviticus 11:47).

Eating pork was condemned.

For behold, the Lord will come with fire and with His chariots, like a whirlwind, to render His anger with fury, and His rebuke with flames of fire. … "Those who sanctify themselves and purify themselves, to go to the gardens after an idol in the midst, eating swine's flesh and the abomination and the mouse, shall be consumed together," says the Lord. (Isaiah 66:15, 17)

Texts on Diet

Therefore, whether you eat or drink, or whatever you do, do all to the glory of God. (1 Corinthians 10:31)

Therefore I urge you to take nourishment, for this is for your survival, since not a hair will fall from the head of any of you. (Acts 27:34)

Texts on Vegetarian Diet

The original diet.

> And God said, "See, I have given you every herb that yields seed which is on the face of all the earth, and every tree whose fruit yields seed; to you it shall be for food. (Genesis 1:29)

Daniel and his friends were vegetarians.

> And the king appointed for them a daily provision of the king's delicacies and of the wine which he drank, and three years of training for them, so that at the end of *that time* they might serve before the king.

> Now from among those of the sons of Judah were Daniel, Hananiah, Mishael, and Azariah.

> To them the chief of the eunuchs gave names: he gave Daniel *the name* Belteshazzar; to Hananiah, Shadrach; to Mishael, Meshach; and to Azariah, Abed-Nego.

> But Daniel purposed in his heart that he would not defile himself with the portion of the king's delicacies, nor with the wine which he drank; therefore he requested of the chief of the eunuchs that he might not defile himself.

> Now God had brought Daniel into the favor and goodwill of the chief of the eunuchs.

> And the chief of the eunuchs said to Daniel, "I fear my lord the king, who has appointed your food and drink. For why should he see your faces looking worse than

the young men who *are* your age? Then you would endanger my head before the king."

So Daniel said to the steward whom the chief of the eunuchs had set over Daniel, Hananiah, Mishael, and Azariah,

"Please test your servants for ten days, and let them give us vegetables to eat and water to drink.

Then let our appearance be examined before you, and the appearance of the young men who eat the portion of the king's delicacies; and as you see fit, *so* deal with your servants."

So he consented with them in this matter, and tested them ten days.

And at the end of ten days their features appeared better and fatter in flesh than all the young men who ate the portion of the king's delicacies. (Daniel 1:5–15)

John the Baptist was a vegetarian (locusts were locust beans).

Now John was clothed with camel's hair and with a leather belt around his waist, and he ate locusts and wild honey. (Mark 1:6)

The diet in heaven will be vegetarian. There will be no killing of animals.

They shall not hurt nor destroy in all My holy mountain, for the earth shall be full of the knowledge of the Lord as the waters cover the sea. (Isaiah 11:9)

The animals in heaven will live peacefully with each other and will be vegetarian.

> The wolf also shall dwell with the lamb, the leopard shall lie down with the young goat, the calf and the young lion and the fatling together; and a little child shall lead them. The cow and the bear shall graze; their young ones shall lie down together; and the lion shall eat straw like the ox. (Isaiah 11:6–7)

Texts on Exercise

> She girds herself with strength, and strengthens her arms. (Proverbs 31:17)

> For bodily exercise profits a little, but godliness is profitable for all things, having promise of the life that now is and of that which is to come. (1 Timothy 4:8)

Texts on Healing

> So you shall serve the Lord your God, and He will bless your bread and your water. And I will take sickness away from the midst of you. (Exodus 23:25)

> Heal the sick, cleanse the lepers, raise the dead, cast out demons. Freely you have received, freely give. (Matthew 10:8)

> "For I will restore health to you and heal you of your wounds," says the Lord, "because they called you an outcast saying: 'This is Zion; no one seeks her.'" (Jeremiah 30:17)

Behold, I will bring it health and healing; I will heal them and reveal to them the abundance of peace and truth. (Jeremiah 33:6)

If you diligently heed the voice of the Lord your God and do what is right in His sight, give ear to His commandments and keep all His statutes, I will put none of the diseases on you which I have brought on the Egyptians. For I am the Lord who heals you. (Exodus 15:26)

When Jesus heard that, He said to them, "Those who are well have no need of a physician, but those who are sick." (Matthew 9:12)

Bless the Lord, O my soul, and forget not all His benefits:
Who forgives all your iniquities, Who heals all your diseases. (Psalm 103:2–3)

Then it shall come to pass, because you listen to these judgments, and keep and do them, that the Lord your God will keep with you the covenant and the mercy which He swore to your fathers.

And He will love you and bless you and multiply you; He will also bless the fruit of your womb and the fruit of your land, your grain and your new wine and your oil, the increase of your cattle and the offspring of your flock, in the land of which He swore to your fathers to give you. You shall be blessed above all peoples; there shall not be a male or female barren among you or among your livestock. And the Lord will take away from you all sickness, and will afflict you with none of the terrible diseases of Egypt which you have

known, but will lay them on all those who hate you."
(Deuteronomy 7:12–15)

Texts on Mental Health

Therefore remove sorrow from your heart, and put away evil from your flesh, for childhood and youth are vanity. (Ecclesiastes 11:10)

Be anxious for nothing, but in everything by prayer and supplication, with thanksgiving, let your requests be made known to God; and the peace of God, which surpasses all understanding, will guard your hearts and minds through Christ Jesus. (Philippians 4:6–7)

There is one who speaks like the piercings of a sword, but the tongue of the wise promotes health. (Proverbs 12:18)

Hope deferred makes the heart sick, but when the desire comes, it is a tree of life. (Proverbs 13:12)

Pleasant words are like a honeycomb, sweetness to the soul and health to the bones. (Proverbs 16:24)

A merry heart does good, like medicine, but a broken spirit dries the bones. (Proverbs 17:22)

Do not be wise in your own eyes; fear the Lord and depart from evil. It will be health to your flesh, and strength to your bones. (Proverbs 3:7–8)

He heals the brokenhearted and binds up their wounds. (Psalm 147:3)

Texts on the Tree of Life

He who has an ear, let him hear what the Spirit says to the churches. To him who overcomes I will give to eat from the tree of life, which is in the midst of the Paradise of God. (Revelation 2:7)

Blessed are those who do His commandments, that they may have the right to the tree of life, and may enter through the gates into the city. (Revelation 22:14)

Texts on Water

And he showed me a pure river of water of life, clear as crystal, proceeding from the throne of God and of the Lamb. (Revelation 22:1)

ABOUT THE AUTHOR

Elvin Adams, MD, MPH, is a graduate of Loma Linda University School of Medicine and holds a master's degree from the Johns Hopkins Bloomberg School of Public Health. He is a specialist certified by the American Board of Internal Medicine and is a fellow of the American College of Preventive Medicine. Adams has also been certified as an HIV/AIDS specialist by the American Academy of HIV Medicine.

Dr. Adams actively promotes those positive health practices that lead to good health and a long life. But he only advocates principles that have been demonstrated to be valid by carefully constructed studies of human populations that are published in peer-reviewed scientific publications.

Adams is the creator of the Best Weigh Nutrition and Weight Management Program and is the author of several books on healthful living. He and his wife have raised three daughters and live in Wilmington, North Carolina.

Printed in the United States
By Bookmasters